RELIEVING NEUROPATHY WITH RESTORE: YOUR ULTIMATE GUIDE TO CONQUERING NEUROPATHY

Dr. David Landry, D.C.
Relieving Neuropathy With RESTORE: Your Ultimate Guide to
Conquering Neuropathy

Published by Spines
ISBN: 979-8-89569-997-3

RELIEVING NEUROPATHY WITH RESTORE: YOUR ULTIMATE GUIDE TO CONQUERING NEUROPATHY

DR. DAVID LANDRY, D.C.

GET ACCESS TO YOUR
FREE REVERSING NEUROPATHY
GIFTS BELOW

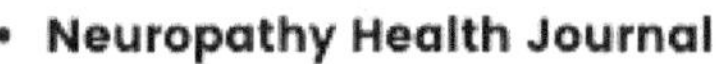

- Neuropathy Health Journal
- Reversing Neuropathy Guide
- 25 Anti-Inflammatory Recipes
- Nerve Damage Quiz
- Free Health Masterclass
- 30-Day Nutrition Plan
- Neuropathy Relief Handbook

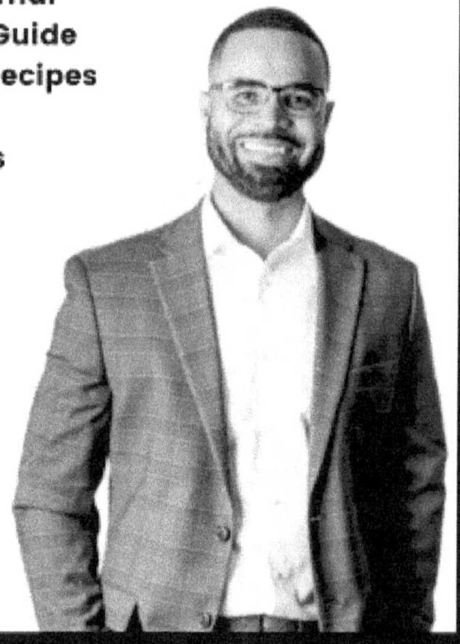

SCAN ME   **DR. DAVID LANDRY DC**

CONTENTS

FOREWORD

Neuropathy is a silent thief, robbing millions of their quality of life, their independence, and their joy. But it doesn't have to be a life sentence. In these pages, you'll discover a powerful weapon against this relentless foe, a guide to reclaiming your well-being, and a community ready to stand beside you on your journey to recovery.

Dr. David Landry, D.C., a true innovator in the field of chiropractic care and a passionate advocate for neuropathy sufferers, has poured his heart and soul into this comprehensive guide. "Relieving Neuropathy With RESTORE: Your Ultimate Guide to Conquering Neuropathy" is not just a book; it's a lifeline, a roadmap, and a testament to the transformative potential of the RESTORE Neuropathy Program.

As a fellow practitioner and a Driven Doc member at The Data Driven Practice, I've had the privilege of witnessing firsthand the remarkable results Dr. Landry and his team have achieved. Their dedication to patient care, their relentless pursuit of knowledge, and their unwavering belief in the power of the human body to heal are truly inspiring.

In this book, Dr. Landry generously shares his wealth of knowledge and experience, demystifying the complexities of neuropathy and empowering readers to take control of their health. The RESTORE Neuropathy Program, meticulously developed and refined over years of clinical practice, offers a holistic and evidence-based approach to managing and relieving neuropathy symptoms.

But "Relieving Neuropathy With RESTORE"" is more than just a collection of techniques and protocols. It's a story of hope, resilience, and the unwavering determination to overcome adversity. Dr. Landry and his team at Optimal Performance Chiropractic are not just practitioners; they are partners, cheerleaders, and guides on your path to pain-free living.

Within these pages, you'll find the tools, knowledge, and support you need to embark on your own transformative journey. Let this book be your companion, your inspiration, and your catalyst for change. Your path to a brighter, pain-free future begins now.

Sincerely,

Dr. Cory Frogley, D.C.

The Data Driven Practice

DISCLAIMER

Disclaimer: The information provided in this book is intended for educational purposes only and is not a substitute for professional medical advice. The author and publisher are not liable for any adverse effects or consequences resulting from the use of the information presented herein. Always consult your physician or a qualified healthcare provider regarding any health concerns or before making any decisions related to your health or treatment.

Results may vary based on individual conditions and compliance with the recommended care plan. The included testimonials are genuine and reflect individual patient experiences but do not guarantee specific results. The services offered in this consultation are for assessment purposes only and do not guarantee treatment or outcome. No claims of superiority or exclusivity are made regarding the services provided. Fees, if advertised, are fully transparent with no hidden conditions. Please consult with Dr. David Landry, D.C. for a personalized assessment of your health condition. This book is not a substitute for professional medical advice.

ABOUT THE AUTHOR

From a young age, I've always been passionate about making a positive impact on people's lives. This drive led me to pursue a career as a Chiropractor, where I realized my potential to help individuals achieve greater health and well-being.

My journey started at California Baptist University, where I earned my Bachelor of Science in Kinesiology. This strong foundation propelled me to Northwestern Health Science University, where I graduated with my Doctorate in Chiropractic in 2009.

My commitment to service then took me on an extraordinary adventure to Peru. For three years, I immersed myself in the vibrant Peruvian culture, becoming fluent in Spanish and sharing the transformative power of chiropractic care through local and national media appearances. I even had the privilege of treating some of Peru's most renowned surfers.

Now, I'm excited to share my passion for helping people achieve optimal health with my hometown community of Riverside. My goal is to empower those suffering from peripheral neuropathy, guiding them towards a pain-free life through the innovative strategies outlined in my book, "Relieving Neuropathy With RESTORE: Your Ultimate Guide to Conquering Neuropathy".

Dr. David Martin Landry II, D.C.

1

NEUROPATHY: THE INVISIBLE EPIDEMIC

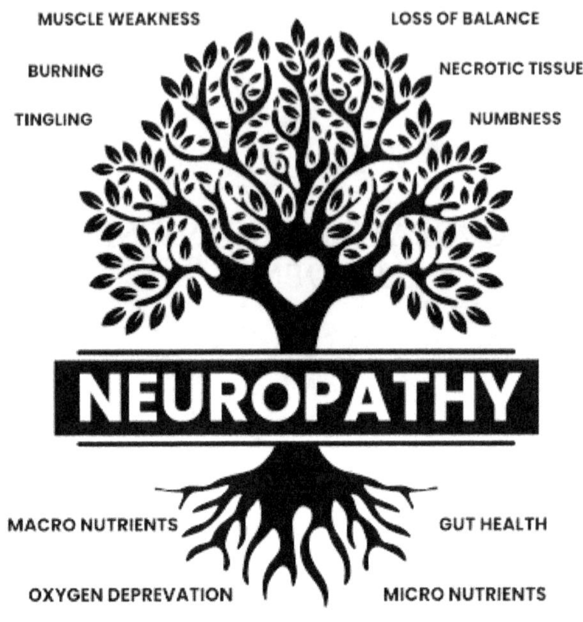

I'll never forget the day Ernie walked into my office, a shadow of his former self. The vibrant energy I'd heard so much about was dimmed, replaced by a weariness that spoke volumes. He told me about the restless legs, the numbness creeping down his right leg, a sensation so profound he couldn't even feel the pedals in his car. His words hung heavy in the air: "Doc, it's like my leg's gone to sleep... and it just won't wake up."

Eight weeks later, a different Ernie stood before me, a grin splitting his face. The spark had returned, his eyes alive with hope. "The numbness is gone, Doc! Almost back to normal. A few more treatments and I'm hitting the road!" His joy was infectious, a testament to the power of the human body to heal, given the right support. Of course, Ernie's experience is his own, and individual results can vary. But it illustrates the profound impact that addressing the root cause of neuropathy can have, rather than simply masking symptoms.

Picture this: It's summertime in California, and the scenery is beautiful. Out of all of the greenery, you notice a tree that appears to be dying: its leaves might be wilting, discolored, or falling off prematurely. While these are the visible symptoms, they are not the root cause of the tree's distress.

You could spray-paint the leaves green, or tape them back on the tree. That appears to fix the problem, right? Of course not. Doing that only masks the symptoms and does not address the root cause of why the tree is dysfunctional.

The underlying issue often lies hidden in the roots. Just as the roots are the tree's lifeline, drawing nutrients and water from the soil to sustain the whole organism, our body's roots — our nervous system — require proper nutrition and care to thrive.

Peripheral neuropathy can be likened to the tree's plight. The symptoms — pain, tingling, numbness, and weakness — are akin to the dying leaves, signaling distress. However, these symptoms are merely the manifestations of deeper issues. The real cause, much like with the tree, lies in the "roots" of our nervous system.

Factors such as systemic diseases, exposure to toxins, infections, or inherited conditions can disrupt the vital flow of nutrients and energy to our nerves, leading to the development of neuropathy. Trying to cover up neuropathy with medications is the same as spray painting leaves or taping them back to the tree- it doesn't address the real problem.

Addressing neuropathy effectively, therefore, requires a holistic approach that nurtures the "roots" — our nervous system — to promote healing and vitality from the inside out. In simpler terms, a holistic approach means treating the whole you, not just the symptoms. It considers how different aspects of your life – your diet, stress levels, sleep patterns – can all work together to influence your neuropathy and your overall health. By addressing these various factors, you can create a personalized plan to manage your neuropathy and reclaim your quality of life.

This is the essence of our RESTORE framework, which focuses on specialization, support, inflammation reduction, regaining function, and tissue regeneration, aiming to restore the body's inherent capacity to heal, much like nourishing the roots to revive a withering tree.

Understanding Neuropathy - The Invisible Pain

Neuropathy is a complex condition that can affect your peripheral nerves, causing them to malfunction due to damage or destruction. It's like having a kink in the wiring of your home, which may not be noticeable at first, but it can eventually lead to a complete blackout.

Similarly, these nerves control critical functions in your body, connecting your brain to your legs, arms, and internal organs—literally every part of you. When they're out of order, you're dealing with not just localized pain; it's a systemic shutdown that can have serious consequences.

This systemic shutdown can have far-reaching implications, impacting every aspect of your daily life. Simple tasks like walking, holding objects, or even digesting food can become complex challenges. The effects extend beyond the physical realm, permeating into your emotional and mental well-being.

Imagine the frustration of not being able to lace up your shoes for a leisurely stroll or the helplessness of struggling to pick up a cherished book. This is the harsh reality faced by countless individuals battling neuropathy. It's a condition that demands attention, understanding, and effective intervention.

Think of your nerves as the electrical wiring in a classic car. Over time, without proper care, those wires can fray or even break. Now, imagine that car trying to win a race with damaged wiring. It might sputter, stall, or even stop altogether.

Your body is no different. If you don't attend to your nerves, your quality of life can stall. You might miss out on the 'race' of life, unable to enjoy activities, outings, or even simple walks in the park.

For example, Sarah, a 55-year-old avid gardener, came to us because she couldn't feel her feet due to neuropathy. She was once active and loved the outdoors, but her condition had reduced her life to watching TV and reading within four walls. And Sarah is not alone; millions face this issue daily.

It's important to recognize that ignoring neuropathy can lead to a worsening of symptoms over time. The impact of neuropathy extends beyond the physical, often affecting emotional well-being, mental health, and social interactions. The challenges of performing daily tasks can lead to feelings of frustration and limitations in daily life.

However, taking a proactive approach to managing neuropathy offers hope for improvement. With timely intervention and a comprehensive approach, many individuals experience a reduction in pain and other symptoms, potentially leading to greater comfort and improved quality of life.

What Causes Neuropathy?

There are many different causes of neuropathy. Some of the most common causes include:

Diabetes

Diabetes is a chronic condition that affects how your body regulates blood sugar (glucose). When blood sugar levels become chronically elevated, it can damage various organs and tissues, including your nerves. This nerve damage is a major contributor to neuropathy.

Here's a breakdown of the main types of diabetes:

- **Type 1 Diabetes:** This autoimmune disease occurs when your body attacks the cells in your pancreas that produce insulin. Insulin is a hormone crucial for unlocking your cells and allowing them to absorb sugar from the bloodstream. Without enough insulin, sugar builds up in the blood, leading to the hallmark symptoms of diabetes.

- **Type 2 Diabetes:** This is the most common form of diabetes. In type 2 diabetes, your body either develops resistance to insulin's effects, or it doesn't produce enough insulin. This also leads to high blood sugar levels.
- **Gestational Diabetes:** This form of diabetes develops during pregnancy and usually resolves after childbirth. However, it can increase your risk of developing type 2 diabetes later in life.

If you're concerned about your risk of diabetes or neuropathy, a crucial first step is to check your blood sugar levels. Early detection and management of diabetes are essential to prevent complications like nerve damage. Here's how you can get started:

- **Talk to your doctor:** Discuss your risk factors and symptoms. They can advise you on the best approach for testing your blood sugar.
- **Consider home blood sugar monitoring:** With your doctor's guidance, you might use a

glucometer, a small device that allows you to easily check your blood sugar levels at home.

- **Start with small changes**: If your blood sugar levels are elevated, even minor adjustments to your diet and lifestyle can make a significant difference.

Remember, early detection and management are key. By taking charge of your blood sugar health, you can significantly reduce your risk of complications like neuropathy. The RESTORE program will be right here to support you every step of the way, providing resources and guidance to empower you on your journey towards optimal health.

Alcoholism

Chronic alcohol consumption is a significant risk factor for neuropathy. Alcohol damages your nerves in two main ways:

- **Direct Toxicity**: Alcohol itself is a neurotoxin, meaning it can directly damage the structure and function of your nerve cells. Imagine your nerves as delicate communication cables. Excessive alcohol acts like a poison, disrupting the signals traveling through these cables, leading to symptoms like numbness, tingling, and weakness.

- **Indirect Damage:** Alcohol disrupts the blood supply to your nerves. Think of your nerves like intricate electrical circuits. Healthy blood flow is crucial for delivering oxygen and essential nutrients to keep these circuits functioning properly. Alcohol damages the delicate lining of blood vessels, leading to restricted blood flow and depriving your nerves of the vital resources they need to thrive. This lack of oxygen and nutrients further contributes to nerve damage.

Excessive alcohol consumption also depletes your body's B vitamins, particularly B1 (thiamine) and B12. These B vitamins play a critical role in nerve health and function. Deficiencies in these vitamins can worsen neuropathy symptoms and lead to a condition called Wernicke-Korsakoff syndrome, known for causing memory problems, balance issues, and severe nerve damage.

If you're concerned about alcohol consumption and its impact on your nerves, the good news is that there's hope. Reducing or eliminating alcohol intake can significantly improve nerve health and potentially reverse some of the damage caused by alcohol.

Vitamin B12 deficiency

Vitamin B12 deficiency is a surprisingly common culprit behind neuropathy. This essential vitamin plays a critical role in maintaining the health and function of your nervous system. Here's how a B12 deficiency can contribute to nerve damage:

- **Protecting the Myelin Sheath:** Imagine your nerves as electrical wires. The myelin sheath acts like a fatty insulating layer surrounding these wires. It protects them and ensures smooth transmission of nerve signals. Vitamin B12 is crucial for the production and maintenance of this myelin sheath. When B12 levels are low, the myelin sheath becomes damaged, exposing the nerves and leaving them vulnerable to injury. This damage disrupts nerve signals, leading to symptoms like numbness, tingling, weakness, and pain.
- **B12 and Nerve Regeneration:** Beyond protection, vitamin B12 is also involved in nerve cell regeneration and repair. A deficiency can hinder your body's ability to repair damaged nerves, further worsening neuropathy symptoms.

So who's most at risk? Certain factors increase your risk of developing a B12 deficiency:

- **Diet**: Strict vegetarians and vegans are at higher risk, as B12 is naturally found in animal products like meat, poultry, fish, and eggs.
- **Age**: As we age, our ability to absorb B12 from food can decline.
- **Digestive Issues**: Conditions like Crohn's disease or pernicious anemia can interfere with B12 absorption.

If you suspect a B12 deficiency, a doctor can perform a simple blood test to confirm it. Treatment typically involves B12 supplements, which can be taken orally or through injections.

For those who can consume animal products, incorporating these B12-rich foods into your diet can be beneficial:

- Meat, poultry, and fish
- Eggs
- Dairy products
- Fortified foods like some cereals and nutritional yeast

Remember: Always consult a doctor before starting any new supplements, especially if you have any underlying health conditions or are taking medications. The RESTORE program recognizes the importance of addressing B12 deficiency as part of our comprehensive approach to neuropathy management.

Autoimmune diseases

Autoimmune diseases are a group of conditions where your body's immune system, normally tasked with fighting off invaders like bacteria and viruses, mistakenly identifies healthy tissues as a threat. In some cases, this misplaced attack can target your nerves, leading to neuropathy. Here's a closer look at how autoimmune diseases can damage your nervous system:

- Certain autoimmune diseases, like Guillain-Barré syndrome and chronic inflammatory demyelinating polyneuropathy (CIDP), directly attack the nerves themselves. This attack can damage the myelin sheath, the protective layer surrounding nerves, or the nerves themselves. This disrupts nerve signaling, causing symptoms like weakness, numbness, tingling, and pain.
- Many autoimmune diseases involve chronic inflammation, a cellular firestorm that

damages surrounding tissues. When nerves are caught in the crossfire of this inflammation, it can lead to nerve damage and neuropathy symptoms.

Examples of Autoimmune Diseases Affecting Nerves:

- **Guillain-Barré Syndrome (GBS):** A rapid onset of muscle weakness, often starting in the legs and spreading upwards, is a hallmark of GBS. This is caused by the immune system attacking the myelin sheath of peripheral nerves.
- **Chronic Inflammatory Demyelinating Polyneuropathy (CIDP):** Similar to GBS, but with a more gradual progression of weakness, numbness, and tingling.
- **Sjogren's Syndrome:** An autoimmune disease affecting the moisture-producing glands in your eyes and mouth. Some people with Sjogren's syndrome also experience neuropathy, likely due to damage to the small nerves in their hands and feet.
- **Lupus:** This systemic autoimmune disease can affect various organs, including the nervous system. Lupus-related neuropathy can cause a

variety of symptoms, depending on which nerves are affected.

If you have an autoimmune disease and experience any symptoms of neuropathy, it's crucial to seek medical attention promptly. Early diagnosis and treatment of the underlying autoimmune condition can help prevent further nerve damage and improve your quality of life.

Infections

Infections caused by viruses, bacteria, and even parasites can be surprising culprits behind neuropathy. These invaders can damage nerves directly or indirectly, leading to a range of symptoms like numbness, tingling, weakness, and pain. Here's a closer look at how infections can wreak havoc on your nervous system:

- Some infections, like Lyme disease caused by bacteria and shingles caused by the varicella-zoster virus (the same virus that causes chickenpox), directly target and damage nerve tissue. In the case of shingles, the virus can travel along nerve pathways, causing the characteristic painful rash and damaging the nerves themselves.

- Many infections trigger a robust immune response, leading to widespread inflammation. While this inflammation helps fight the infection, it can also damage surrounding tissues, including nerves. This collateral damage can disrupt nerve function and contribute to neuropathy symptoms.

Common Infectious Causes of Neuropathy:

- **Lyme disease:** This tick-borne illness can cause a variety of neurological symptoms, including neuropathy. The bacteria responsible for Lyme disease can directly infiltrate nerve tissue and cause inflammation, leading to nerve damage. Early diagnosis and treatment of Lyme disease are crucial to prevent long-term nerve damage.
- **Shingles:** This painful condition, characterized by a blistering rash, can also cause neuropathy. The varicella-zoster virus can travel along nerve pathways, damaging them and causing pain, numbness, and weakness in the affected area. Even after the rash clears, post-herpetic neuralgia, a form of neuropathy, can persist for months or even years.
- **HIV/AIDS:** The human immunodeficiency virus (HIV) can damage the nervous system in

various ways, including causing neuropathy. HIV can directly infect nerve cells or indirectly damage them through the inflammatory response it triggers. Early diagnosis and treatment of HIV can help prevent or slow the progression of nerve damage.

- Other Infections: While less common, other infections like **cytomegalovirus (CMV)**, **Epstein-Barr virus (EBV)**, and some bacterial infections can also cause neuropathy.

If you suspect you might have an infection and experience symptoms of neuropathy, seeking prompt medical attention is crucial. Early diagnosis and treatment of the underlying infection can help prevent further nerve damage and improve your long-term prognosis.

Medications

Medications play a vital role in treating various health conditions, but some can damage nerves directly or indirectly, leading to symptoms like numbness, tingling, weakness, and pain. Here's a breakdown of how certain medications can contribute to neuropathy:

- Chemotherapy drugs used to fight cancer are a prime example. These powerful medications work by targeting rapidly dividing cells, unfortunately, some nerve cells can be caught in the crossfire. This damage to the nerve cells' DNA can lead to neuropathy.

- Certain antibiotics, particularly those from the class known as fluoroquinolones, can disrupt the production of myelin, the protective sheath surrounding nerves. This lack of myelin leaves the nerves vulnerable to damage and can contribute to neuropathy symptoms.

Medications that can cause neuropathy:

- **Chemotherapy drugs:** These potent drugs used to treat cancer are a well-known cause of neuropathy. The specific type of chemotherapy drug and dosage can influence the risk and severity of neuropathy.
- **Antibiotics:** While uncommon, fluoroquinolone antibiotics like Ciprofloxacin (Cipro) have been associated with neuropathy.
- **Anticonvulsants:** Medications used to control seizures, like Gabapentin and Pregabalin, can sometimes cause numbness, tingling, or weakness as a side effect. This doesn't necessarily indicate neuropathy, but it's

important to discuss these sensations with your doctor.

- **Pain medications**: Certain chronic pain medications, like Tricyclic antidepressants (TCAs) and some opioids, can cause numbness or tingling as a side effect.

Medications can be lifesavers, but it's crucial to weigh the benefits against potential side effects like neuropathy.

Physical injuries

Accidents happen, and sometimes those accidents can leave a lasting impact on your nervous system. Physical injuries, from car accidents and falls to sports injuries and repetitive stress, can be a significant cause of neuropathy. Here's how these injuries contribute to nerve damage:

- **Direct Nerve Compression or Laceration:** The most obvious scenario is a direct blow to a nerve. A car accident, fall, or even a deep cut can severely damage or sever a nerve, leading to immediate symptoms like numbness, weakness, and pain in the affected area.
- **Stretched or Pinched Nerves:** Even less dramatic injuries can cause neuropathy.

Repetitive stress injuries, like carpal tunnel syndrome, occur when a nerve gets compressed or pinched by surrounding tissues. Over time, this compression can disrupt nerve function and lead to symptoms like tingling, numbness, and weakness.

- **Blood Vessel Damage and Starved Nerves:** Physical injuries can also damage blood vessels supplying nerves. These blood vessels deliver oxygen and essential nutrients to keep nerves healthy. If these blood vessels are damaged, the nerves become starved of these vital resources, leading to nerve dysfunction and potential neuropathy symptoms.

Examples of injuries leading to neuropathy:

- **Car accidents:** The force of a car accident can cause various injuries, including nerve damage. This can range from mild compression to complete nerve severance, depending on the severity of the accident.
- **Falls:** A fall, especially on an outstretched hand, can damage nerves in the wrist or arm. This can lead to carpal tunnel syndrome or other types of neuropathy.

- **Sports injuries:** Repetitive stress from certain sports can compress nerves, leading to neuropathy. For example, carpal tunnel syndrome is common in athletes who grip objects repeatedly, like cyclists and weightlifters.
- **Surgery:** While surgery is often necessary, it can sometimes damage nerves during the procedure. This can lead to post-surgical neuropathy, causing numbness, pain, or weakness in the affected area.

If you experience an injury and develop symptoms like numbness, tingling, or weakness, seeking medical attention promptly is crucial. Early diagnosis and treatment of nerve damage can minimize long-term complications and improve your recovery.

Idiopathic neuropathy

Neuropathy can be like a detective story – sometimes the culprit is clear, but other times, the cause remains a puzzling mystery. Idiopathic neuropathy falls into this category. It refers to nerve damage where, despite extensive evaluation, no underlying reason can be identified. While idiopathic neuropathy is considered uncommon, it can be a significant source of frustration for those affected.

Here's a closer look at this enigmatic form of neuropathy:

- **Ruling Out the Usual Suspects:** Extensive testing for common causes like diabetes, vitamin deficiencies, autoimmune diseases, and infections is usually conducted. If all these come back negative, then idiopathic neuropathy becomes a possibility.
- **Not a Hallmark of Rarity:** While uncommon, idiopathic neuropathy isn't exceptionally rare. It affects a significant portion of neuropathy cases, making it an important piece of the neuropathy puzzle.

Even though the exact cause of idiopathic neuropathy remains elusive, there's still hope. Here's why:

- **Focus on What You Can Control:** While the cause might be a mystery, the focus can shift to managing symptoms and improving your quality of life. This can involve lifestyle modifications, targeted supplements, and pain management strategies.
- **Research on the Horizon:** Scientists continue to delve deeper into the potential causes of idiopathic neuropathy. Advances in research

might someday shed light on the underlying mechanisms and lead to more targeted treatments.

The RESTORE program acknowledges the challenges of navigating idiopathic neuropathy. We'll explore various strategies to support your nervous system health and empower you to become an active participant in your own wellness journey, even in the face of uncertainty.

If you have any of the risk factors for neuropathy, it's important to talk to your doctor about ways to reduce your risk of developing the condition. At Optimal Performance Chiropractic, we have personalized, holistic treatments available to help you manage the symptoms of neuropathy and improve your quality of life.

What are the Symptoms of Neuropathy?

The symptoms of neuropathy vary depending on the type of neuropathy and the affected nerves. However, some of the most common symptoms of neuropathy include:

- **Numbness and tingling**: Numbness and tingling are often the first symptoms of neuropathy. They usually start in the fingertips or toes and gradually spread up the arms or legs.

- **Pain:** Neuropathy can cause various types of pain, including burning, stabbing, and shooting pain. The pain is often worse at night and may be accompanied by a feeling of coldness or heat in the affected area.
- **Weakness:** Neuropathy can cause muscle weakness in the affected area, making it difficult to walk, climb stairs, or lift objects.
- **Loss of coordination and balance:** Neuropathy can cause loss of coordination and balance, increasing the risk of falls.
- **Autonomic symptoms:** Neuropathy can also affect the autonomic nervous system, which controls the body's involuntary functions, such as heart rate, blood pressure, and digestion. Autonomic symptoms of neuropathy can include:
  - Changes in heart rate or blood pressure
  - Difficulty digesting food
  - Difficulty urinating or having bowel movements
  - Changes in sweating patterns
  - Sexual dysfunction

In severe cases, neuropathy can lead to paralysis and loss of sensation in the affected area, making it difficult or impossible to move the affected parts of the body. It can also make it difficult to feel pain, leading to injuries.

If you have severe neuropathy, it's important to see a doctor regularly to monitor your condition and manage any complications. There are treatments available to help slow the progression of neuropathy and relieve the symptoms to improve your quality of life.

Here are some tips for managing severe neuropathy:

- **Get regular medical checkups.** Your doctor will monitor your condition and ensure you get the appropriate treatment.
- **Follow your doctor's treatment program.** This may include supplements, lifestyle & dietary changes, light therapy, nerve stimulation, SoftWave therapy (a non-invasive sound wave treatment for pain and tissue healing), vibration therapy, chiropractic, or other therapies.
- **Take care of your feet.** Neuropathy can make it difficult to feel pain in your feet, leading to injuries. Inspect your feet regularly for any signs of injury or infection.

- **Manage your blood sugar levels.** If you have diabetes (or even if you don't!), it's essential to manage your blood sugar levels as well as possible. Doing so will help to slow the progression of neuropathy.
- **Maintain a healthy weight.** Being overweight or obese can put extra stress on your nerves. Maintaining a healthy weight can help to reduce the risk of neuropathy and improve your overall health.

Navigating the Waves: Effective Coping Strategies for Neuropathy

Living with neuropathy presents a unique set of challenges. The persistent pain, numbness, and other symptoms can significantly impact your daily life, emotional well-being, and overall sense of control. But remember, you're not alone in this journey. Effective coping strategies can empower you to navigate these challenges and maintain a fulfilling life.

Embracing a Holistic Approach:

Coping with neuropathy goes beyond simply managing pain. It's about nurturing your physical, emotional, and mental well-being holistically. Here are some key strategies to help you navigate this journey:

Physical Strategies:

- **Movement is Medicine:** Regular exercise, tailored to your abilities, improves nerve function, reduces pain, and boosts mood. Explore gentle activities like walking, yoga, or tai chi.
- **Rest and Relaxation:** Prioritize adequate sleep and relaxation techniques like meditation or deep breathing to manage stress and promote nerve healing.
- **Nourishing Your Body:** Choose a healthy diet rich in fruits, vegetables, and whole grains to provide essential nutrients for nerve health. Consider consulting a nutritionist for personalized guidance.
- **Alternative Therapies:** Explore complementary therapies like massage, acupuncture, or biofeedback to manage pain and promote relaxation. Discuss these options with your healthcare professional to ensure they are safe and appropriate for your specific case.

Emotional and Mental Strategies:

- **Connecting with Support:** Join a support group or connect with other individuals living with neuropathy. Sharing experiences and fostering emotional connections can provide invaluable support and understanding.
- **Mindfulness and Cognitive Behavioral Therapy (CBT):** These techniques can help you manage stress, negative thoughts, and anxiety associated with neuropathy, fostering resilience and improving coping skills.
- **Gratitude and Positive Thinking:** Cultivating a grateful mindset and focusing on the positive aspects of your life can boost your mood and overall well-being.

Remember:

- **Individualized Approach:** What works for one person might not work for another. Experiment and find the strategies that resonate most with you.
- **Open Communication:** Maintain open communication with your healthcare professional. Discuss your specific challenges and concerns, and work together to create a

> personalized treatment plan that addresses your physical, emotional, and mental needs.

- **Empowerment is Key:** Remember, you have the power to manage your neuropathy and live a fulfilling life. Utilize these coping strategies, build a strong support network, and actively participate in your healthcare journey.

By embracing a holistic approach and incorporating these effective coping strategies, you can navigate the challenges of neuropathy with resilience and regain control over your well-being. Remember, you are not alone in this journey.

Revolutionizing Neuropathy Treatment: The RESTORE Healing Framework

At Optimal Performance Chiropractic, our vision is to create a community where people have taken control of their health, where drugs and surgery are a last resort, and where longevity and quality of life go hand-in-hand. We want every child to experience the joys of life without disease or dysfunction and for every individual to live a clear and connected life.

We use state-of-the-art technology and the latest research to bring this vision to life. We offer a new solution for neuropathy pain that combines a drug-free, non-surgical approach with the most advanced neuropathy pain relief technology available, which is our RESTORE healing framework.

And many patients are seeing great results because of this program, even those who have "tried everything" else before. It's a proven process to manage and relieve neuropathy symptoms effectively.

Here's a brief overview of **R.E.S.T.O.R.E:**

R - Remove Toxins

Our bodies can accumulate toxins from the environment, food, and even our own metabolic processes. These toxins can damage our nerves and contribute to neuropathy. My approach starts with identifying and reducing your exposure to harmful substances, giving your body a much-needed detox.

E - Enhance Nutrition

Nerves, like any other part of your body, require the right nutrients to function properly. We'll focus on a diet rich in healing foods that support nerve repair and reduce inflammation. Think of this as supercharging your nerves with the building blocks they need.

S - Stimulate Circulation

Healthy blood flow is essential for delivering oxygen and nutrients to your nerves. We'll work on strategies to improve circulation, ensuring your nerves get the vital resources they need to heal.

T - Transform Habits

Sometimes, our daily habits can unknowingly worsen nerve damage. We'll identify potential factors contributing to your neuropathy and make beneficial adjustments for healthier nerves.

O - Optimize Nerve Function

Through specific therapies and techniques tailored to your needs, we'll aim to optimize the communication and function of your nerves themselves. This will help reduce pain signals and improve overall nerve health.

R - Revitalize Movement

Gentle, targeted movement is crucial for nerve health as it boosts circulation and promotes nerve regeneration. Together, we'll develop an exercise plan that's both safe and effective for you.

E - Encourage Regeneration

Your nerves have an incredible ability to heal, and we'll use a variety of approaches to support this natural process. Through nutrition, targeted therapies, and lifestyle changes, we'll encourage your nerves to regenerate and rebuild.

No matter what your individual needs are, we will work with you to develop a tailored treatment plan that will help you achieve your health goals.

ACTION STEP: Start a daily journal of your symptoms. This will allow you to more accurately sense your level of improvement when starting a neuropathy treatment regimen.

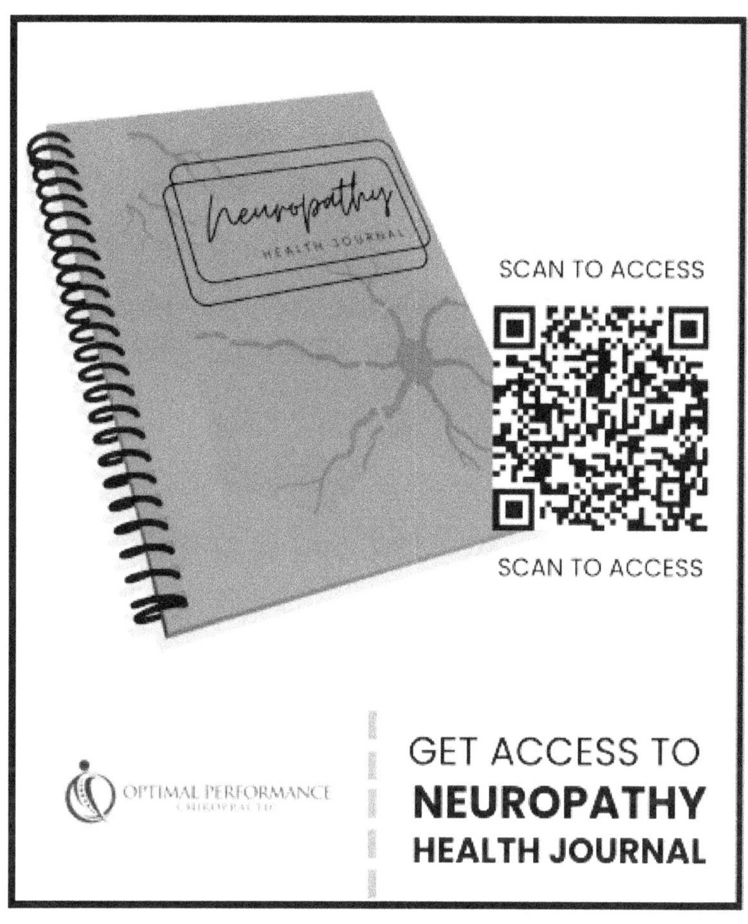

Unlock Your Path to Neuropathy Relief Now: Dial (951) 405-8868 to Speak With Us Today!

2

————

RESTORE: A NEW HOPE FOR NEUROPATHY

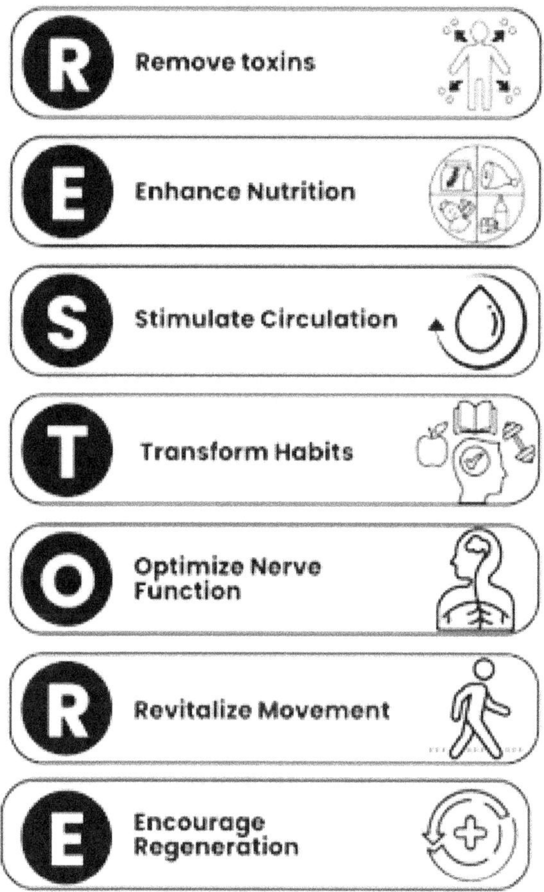

Neuropathy, a condition characterized by nerve damage and often debilitating symptoms, can leave individuals feeling powerless. Traditional treatments often prioritize symptom management through medications, leaving many longing for a more holistic and effective solution.

This chapter introduces the RESTORE program, a beacon of hope for those seeking a path beyond mere pain relief. We'll delve into the limitations of traditional approaches and unveil RESTORE's unique philosophy, built on addressing root causes, personalized care, and non-invasive therapies.

Discover how RESTORE aims not just to manage symptoms, but to truly heal and empower individuals to reclaim a vibrant, pain-free life. Are you ready to explore this transformative approach and unlock the promise of RESTORE? Keep reading and start your journey towards true healing.

The Shortfalls of Traditional Treatments

When you're struggling with neuropathy, it's natural to seek help from your doctor. However, many people find the conventional medical approach to be frustratingly limited. Here's why:

- **Treating the Symptoms, Not the Cause:** Traditional medicine often focuses on masking the pain of neuropathy with medications. While painkillers can offer temporary relief, they do nothing to address the underlying nerve damage causing your symptoms. It's like putting a band-aid on a broken pipe – the problem just gets worse over time.

- **The Risks of Long-Term Medication Use:** Many neuropathy medications come with significant side effects. Painkillers like opioids can be habit-forming, while others can have negative impacts on your stomach, liver, and kidneys. The longer you use them, the higher the risks.

- **A "One-Size-Fits-All" Approach:** There are many different causes of neuropathy – diabetes, chemotherapy, injuries, autoimmune disorders, and more. Yet, conventional treatments often don't adequately differentiate between these root causes. They rely on a few standard drugs or procedures, regardless of your individual situation.

- **Limited Focus on Lifestyle & Prevention:** While lifestyle factors like healthy eating, exercise, and managing underlying health conditions are crucial in neuropathy management, conventional medicine rarely places enough emphasis on these important components. You might get a prescription, but little guidance on the long-term changes that can truly optimize your nerve health.

This isn't to say that all conventional doctors are ineffective in treating neuropathy. However, the limitations of the mainstream system are real, and they explain why many people continue to suffer despite seeking medical help.

Why Traditional Treatments Prioritize Symptom Relief

As a holistic doctor who treats neuropathy, I'm often asked why traditional neuropathy treatments focus on relieving symptoms instead of fixing the underlying cause of the problem. There are a few reasons for this:

- Traditional medicine, like an old sheet of music, often follows a reductionist tune. It dissects the body into separate notes, focusing on individual parts rather than the grand symphony they create together. For acute illnesses, this approach hits the right chords. But when it comes to chronic conditions like neuropathy, it's like playing a solo in a full orchestra—it lacks harmony.

- Neuropathy is a puzzling condition, a tangled web of nerves gone haywire. While modern medicine has made strides, the root causes remain elusive, shrouded in mystery. This means there's no magic bullet, no one-size-fits-all cure. Instead, traditional treatments focus on soothing the symptoms, offering a reprieve from the burning, tingling, or numbing sensations that can make life a daily struggle.

- The healthcare system is driven by profit. Pharmaceutical companies make billions of dollars each year selling prescription medications, including pain medications and other medications used to treat neuropathy symptoms. It is more profitable for the healthcare system to treat symptoms than to cure diseases.

In addition to these reasons, greed plays a role in why traditional neuropathy treatments focus on relieving symptoms instead of fixing the underlying cause of the problem. Pharmaceutical companies have a vested interest in keeping people sick so that they can continue to sell them medications.

The pharmaceutical industry spends more money paying our lawmakers (lobbying) every year than any other industry. This is typically hundreds of millions of dollars per year. Because of this, laws are continually passed that allow major profits to pharmaceutical companies and keep patients as lifelong customers of their drugs.

Pharmaceutical companies also spend billions of dollars each year on advertising to convince people that they need drugs to be healthy. Did you know that the United States is one of only two countries in the entire world that allow pharmaceutical advertising?

The good news is that there are other non-addictive, non-invasive treatments available for neuropathy, such as our RESTORE healing framework that we provide.

Case Studies Where Traditional Treatments Failed

Here are some specific case studies of patients who suffered from peripheral neuropathy and did not find relief or improvement with conventional treatments.

- A 40-year-old woman who suffered from chronic neuropathic pain after a spinal cord injury[1]. She had tried various medications, such as opioids, antidepressants, and anticonvulsants, but none of them provided adequate pain relief or improved her function. She also experienced severe side effects, such as nausea, constipation, drowsiness, and addiction. She was frustrated, hopeless, and suicidal.

- A 50-year-old man who developed diabetic neuropathy and foot ulcers[2]. He had poor glycemic control and did not follow a healthy diet or lifestyle. He had tried various wound care products, such as dressings, creams, and antibiotics, but none of them healed his ulcers or prevented infection. He was at risk of amputation and sepsis. He was terrified, angry, and desperate.
- A 60-year-old woman who had chemotherapy-induced peripheral neuropathy[3]. She had received chemotherapy for ovarian cancer, which caused nerve damage and neuropathic pain in her hands and feet. She had tried various supplements, such as vitamins, antioxidants, and amino acids, but none of them relieved or repaired the nerve damage or reduced the pain. She also experienced fatigue, weakness, and depression. She was devastated, scared, and confused.

Peripheral neuropathy is a challenging condition that can affect the quality of life of many patients. However, conventional treatments are not always effective, safe, or suitable for every case. Therefore, it's important to explore alternative options that can offer more natural, holistic, or innovative solutions for peripheral neuropathy, like the RESTORE neuropathy program. By considering the individual needs, preferences, and goals of each patient, we can find the best option that can help them cope with or overcome peripheral neuropathy.

1: https://www.hindawi.com/journals/nri/2022/8336561/

2: https://link.springer.com/article/10.1007/s11916-022-01061-7

3: https://www.frontiersin.org/articles/10.3389/fendo.2019.00929/full

RESTORE: Elevating Neuropathy Treatment Beyond Symptom Management

The promise of the RESTORE program is quite profound. It offers a comprehensive, multi-faceted approach to not only alleviate neuropathic pain and improve function, but also to promote true healing and a return to a vibrant, pain-free life.

Unlike traditional treatments that often focus solely on symptom management through medications, the RESTORE program delves much deeper. It addresses the root causes of neuropathy, recognizing that it's not just a localized issue but a complex interplay of factors, including blood sugar dynamics, tissue regeneration, nerve rebuilding, and more.

Take tissue regeneration, for instance. Instead of merely masking symptoms, RESTORE aims to stimulate the body's own regenerative capacities. Through innovative therapies like SoftWave and light therapy, we encourage the growth of new blood vessels and nerves, facilitating genuine healing.

Furthermore, the program acknowledges the critical role of balanced blood sugar in nerve health and provides a tailored, holistic approach to address this aspect. By understanding the intricate dance between insulin and glucagon, RESTORE offers a nuanced strategy often overlooked in traditional treatments.

But what truly sets RESTORE apart is its individualized approach. We understand that no two individuals experience neuropathy in the exact same way. By tailoring treatments to each person's unique needs, we increase the likelihood of success and offer a more personalized path to healing.

In essence, the RESTORE program isn't merely about managing symptoms; it seeks to restore, regenerate, and rejuvenate. It's a promise of not just living with neuropathy but thriving beyond it. That's the fundamental difference and the potential game-changer that sets RESTORE apart from conventional neuropathy treatments.

From Despair to Hope: Deborah's Remarkable Neuropathy Recovery

A diagnosis of diabetes brought a wave of new challenges for Deborah, including the relentless pain of neuropathy in her feet. Sleepless nights, ineffective medications, and a bleak prognosis from her doctors left her feeling defeated. The future, once filled with possibilities, seemed to shrink as the threat of worsening symptoms and needing a wheelchair loomed over her.

Then, hope flickered anew. The RESTORE approach offered something different. Within just two weeks, a remarkable transformation had begun. The stabbing pains in Deborah's feet subsided, replaced by the sweet relief of restful nights. Each morning brought a fresh sense of amazement – she'd actually slept.

The despair that had consumed her was replaced by determination. Emboldened by this newfound freedom from pain, Deborah isn't satisfied with merely feeling better. She's eager to embrace all that her recovery holds, her eyes fixed firmly on the future and what else this journey with the Optimal Performance Chiropractic team might bring.

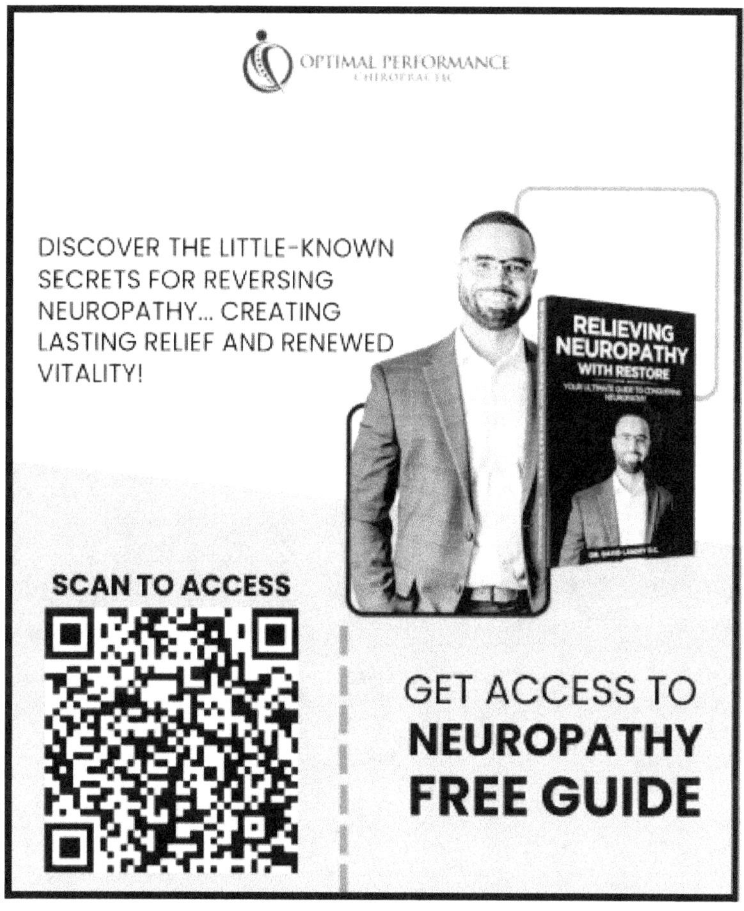

From Painful Nights to Walking a Mile: Susan's Story

"When I first got here at Optimal Performance Chiropractic, I couldn't sleep as well because my feet were hurting quite a bit. I would have to put one of those wedge pillows so my feet would feel better, and then I had a compression stocking constantly on my ankle. I couldn't walk the distance that I wanted to. I would wake up in the middle of the night. My feet would hurt. I would have to get up and flex them for them to stop hurting. But now, I'm not even halfway through the RESTORE program, and I'm already experiencing some phenomenal results. The pain has improved. I'm walking now. I did a mile the other day with my husband."

** This testimonial is not intended to represent typical results.*

Unlock Your Path to Neuropathy Relief Now: Dial (951) 405-8868 to Speak With Us Today!

3

THE PLATE OF PAIN: UNHEALTHY DIET & NERVE DAMAGE

The Typical American Diet and Blood Sugar Imbalance

Something I have come to realize is that factual nutrition classes NEED to be taught in our elementary schools. Have you ever looked at the food that is served to our children across America on a daily basis?

That leads to a question... Have you ever wondered why so many people in the United States suffer from peripheral neuropathy?

The truth is the typical American diet plays a significant role in this condition. When we consume excessive amounts of refined carbohydrates, sugars, and processed foods, we put our blood sugar levels on a roller coaster ride. This can lead to chronic inflammation and oxidative stress, which can damage our nerves and contribute to the development of neuropathy. Here are some common culprits to watch out for:

- **Sugary drinks:** Soda, sports drinks, and fruit juices are loaded with added sugars.
- **Refined carbohydrates:** White bread, pasta, pastries, and white rice are quickly digested, causing blood sugar spikes.
- **Processed meats:** Hot dogs, deli meats, and bacon are often high in sodium and unhealthy fats.
- **Fried foods:** French fries, onion rings, and fried snacks are loaded with unhealthy fats and can contribute to inflammation.
- **Packaged snacks:** Cookies, chips, and crackers are often high in refined carbohydrates, unhealthy fats, and added sodium.

Imagine the American diet as a grand theater, its spotlight trained on a trio of actors: refined carbs, sugars, and processed foods. They pirouette onto the stage, their entrance swift and dazzling. But behind the scenes, a drama unfolds—one that stars our blood sugar levels.

As the curtain rises, our cells applaud. These foods, like eager performers, leap into action. But their swift digestion sends blood sugar soaring—a standing ovation that doesn't last. Enter insulin, the backstage maestro. It cues the exit music, urging sugar out of the limelight. Yet, if this dance repeats too often, our cells become jaded, ignoring insulin's pleas.

Now, let's explore the subplot—the nerves. AGEs, the masked villains, emerge. They're the sticky residue of sugar bonding with proteins, tarnishing nerve cells. It's like caramelized sugar clinging to a saucepan—a stubborn stain.

But there's a twist: the blood vessels—the lifeblood conduits—are also ensnared. High sugar coats their walls, narrowing the passage. Oxygen and nutrients, once delivered with grace, now stutter. It's nerve malnourishment, a silent erosion.

The Dietary Foundation of Neuropathy

The typical American diet is not only high in refined carbohydrates and sugars, but it's also often low in nutrient-rich foods such as fruits, vegetables, and healthy protein sources. These foods contain essential vitamins, minerals, and antioxidants necessary for nerve health.

When we don't consume enough nutrient-rich foods, our nerves are more vulnerable to damage. That's because our bodies can't produce all the nutrients our nerves need to function properly. Here are two case studies that illustrate how the typical American diet negatively impacts blood sugar and nerve health, which has led to neuropathy:

Case Study 1

John was a 55-year-old man who had been diagnosed with type 2 diabetes for ten years. He had a typical American diet high in processed foods, refined carbohydrates, and sugary drinks. He also had a sedentary lifestyle.

Over time, John's blood sugar levels became poorly controlled, leading to damage to his nerves, and he developed neuropathy in his feet and legs. He experienced numbness, tingling, and pain in his feet and legs. He also had difficulty walking and standing.

John's doctor advised him to make changes to his diet and lifestyle. John started eating a healthier diet lower in processed foods, refined carbohydrates, and sugary drinks. He also started exercising regularly.

As a result of these changes, John's blood sugar levels improved significantly. His neuropathy symptoms also improved. He now has less pain and numbness in his feet and legs, and he can walk and stand more easily.

Case Study 2

Mary was a 45-year-old woman who had no known health problems. She ate a typical American diet high in processed foods, refined carbohydrates, and sugary drinks.

One day, Mary started experiencing numbness and tingling in her hands and feet. She also had difficulty walking and standing. She went to see her doctor, who diagnosed her with neuropathy.

Mary's doctor was surprised that she had neuropathy as she had no known risk factors for the condition. However, after reviewing her diet, the doctor realized she consumed too many processed foods, refined carbohydrates, and sugary drinks.

The doctor advised Mary to make changes to her diet. Mary started eating a healthier diet lower in processed foods, refined carbohydrates, and sugary drinks. She also started exercising regularly.

As a result of these changes, Mary's neuropathy symptoms improved significantly. She now has less numbness and tingling in her hands and feet, and she can walk and stand more easily.

These two case studies illustrate how the typical American diet can negatively impact blood sugar and nerve health, leading to neuropathy. By making simple changes to our diet, such as eating more nutrient-rich foods and limiting processed foods, we can help protect our nerves and reduce our risk of developing neuropathy.

Paying attention to specific nutrients that are crucial in maintaining nerve health is also essential. One such group of nutrients is the B vitamins, which are indispensable for the proper functioning of our nerves.

A deficiency in B vitamins can lead to nerve damage and neuropathy, emphasizing the importance of including these vitamins in our diet. Fortunately, B vitamins are readily available in nutrient-rich foods such as whole grains, legumes, nuts, seeds, and high-quality protein sources.

Similarly, another vital nutrient for nerve health is vitamin E. This antioxidant nutrient plays a significant role in safeguarding our cells from damage, including nerve cells. By incorporating vitamin E-rich foods like nuts, seeds, and avocados into our diet, we can provide our nerves with the protection they need to stay healthy and prevent the development of neuropathy.

Gut Health - One of Many Root Causes

Emerging research suggests that an often-overlooked factor in the development of peripheral neuropathy is gut health. The gut, often referred to as the "second brain," plays a crucial role in overall well-being, including the health of the nervous system.

The gut is home to trillions of microbes collectively known as the gut microbiota. These microorganisms contribute to various physiological functions, including the regulation of the immune system and inflammation. Disruptions in the balance of gut bacteria, known as dysbiosis, can trigger an inflammatory response that may contribute to nerve damage and exacerbate peripheral neuropathy.

The gut-brain axis, a bidirectional communication system between the gut and the central nervous system, is implicated in peripheral neuropathy. Imbalances in gut microbiota can influence this axis, leading to systemic inflammation and oxidative stress, both of which are implicated in nerve damage.

Research suggests that addressing gut health through probiotics, prebiotics, and a balanced diet may positively impact peripheral neuropathy symptoms. By recognizing the intricate connection between gut health and peripheral nerves, healthcare professionals and individuals alike can explore holistic approaches to manage and potentially prevent this debilitating condition.

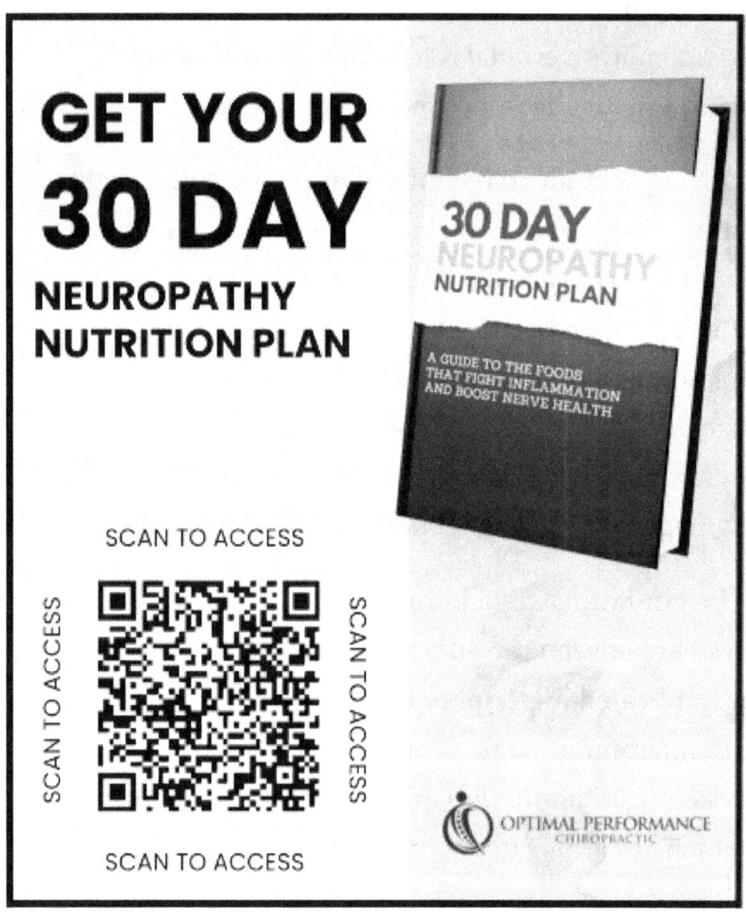

Howard's Journey to Less Pain

"Dr. Landry and the Optimal Performance Chiropractic staff always welcome and take good care of me. They improved my neuropathy in my legs and feet by over

50%. I am so very thankful for finding their office in Riverside."

** Your results may be different.*

Unlock Your Path to Neuropathy Relief Now: Dial (951) 405-8868 to Speak With Us Today!

4

THE BLOOD SUGAR EQUATION: UNLOCKING NERVE HEALTH

The Insulin-Glucagon Balance

Think of insulin as the key that unlocks the door for glucose (sugar) to enter your cells. After you eat a meal, your blood sugar rises, and this signals the pancreas to release insulin. Insulin travels through the bloodstream and attaches to receptors on cells throughout the body, especially muscle, liver, and fat cells. This attachment triggers cells to open up and take in glucose for energy or storage.

How Insulin Relates to Neuropathy

High blood sugar (hyperglycemia), as we've discussed, is a major culprit in nerve damage. Over time, chronically high blood sugar leads to direct damage to nerves through processes like glycation (the formation of harmful AGEs) and the disruption of metabolic pathways within nerve cells.

Insulin, like a diligent traffic cop, works to keep blood sugar levels in a safe range. After a meal, it ensures that glucose is efficiently escorted out of the bloodstream and into cells, preventing prolonged spikes. The less time your blood sugar spends at high levels, the lower your risk of direct nerve damage.

Supporting Nerve Health: Fueling Optimal Function

Nerves, like all cells in your body, require a constant supply of glucose for energy. Think of glucose as their fuel source. Insulin acts like a delivery service, ensuring that this fuel reaches nerves and allows them to operate effectively.

Nerve functions include transmitting signals for the sensations of touch, pain, and temperature. Additionally, they help control other bodily processes, such as muscle movement and balance. When insulin isn't functioning properly, or when nerves become less sensitive to insulin, this vital fuel delivery system is compromised. Nerves that are starved for glucose struggle to function optimally, potentially leading to the symptoms of neuropathy.

Glucagon: The Blood Sugar Stabilizer

While insulin's role is to lower blood sugar, glucagon's primary duty is to raise it when levels fall too low. This often happens between meals, overnight while you sleep, or during prolonged periods of exercise when your body's energy stores are getting depleted.

Think of your liver as a glucose storage pantry. When your blood sugar dips, glucagon acts as the key that unlocks this pantry. Glucagon signals the liver to break down stored glucose (called glycogen) and release it into the bloodstream, providing a quick boost to bring your blood sugar levels back up to a normal range.

Glucagon's Connection to Neuropathy

While glucagon's primary function is ensuring you have enough available glucose for energy, this delicate balance can be disrupted in several ways that impact neuropathy risk:

- **Insulin Resistance:** In insulin resistance, even with normal glucagon function, the liver becomes less responsive to its signal to release glucose. This can contribute to low blood sugar (hypoglycemia), especially if someone on medication for diabetes miscalculates a dose or skips a meal. While less directly damaging to nerves than chronic high blood sugar, frequent drops in blood sugar can still be harmful over the long term.

- **Impaired Glucagon Response:** In some advanced cases of diabetes, the ability to produce sufficient glucagon can be compromised. This can lead to severe hypoglycemia (dangerously low blood sugar), increasing the risk of complications, some of which can themselves affect the nerves.

The Importance of the Glucagon Safety Net

Glucagon provides a crucial safety mechanism to prevent serious drops in blood sugar. It works hand-in-hand with insulin to maintain balance and ensure a steady supply of glucose for your body's energy needs, including those of your nerves.

The Delicate Dance: Insulin and Glucagon

Insulin and glucagon work in a constant see-saw fashion to maintain your blood sugar within a narrow, healthy range. This delicate equilibrium is essential for optimal health and plays a vital role in protecting your nerves. Imbalances in insulin/glucagon function can disrupt blood sugar levels, contributing to neuropathy development.

Preventing Neuropathy: The Importance of Balance

A well-functioning insulin-glucagon system is indispensable for neuropathy prevention. When insulin works effectively, cells respond to its signal, readily absorbing glucose from the blood. This keeps blood sugar levels stable and prevents nerve damage. On the other hand, when cells become resistant to insulin, your blood sugar levels remain consistently high, increasing the risk for neuropathy and its associated complications.

The dynamic balance between insulin and glucagon is crucial for maintaining healthy blood sugar levels and thus protecting nerves from damage. Insulin works to lower blood sugar and provide nerves with energy, while glucagon serves as a counterbalance, raising blood sugar when levels dip too low. Understanding the delicate interplay of these hormones is key to grasping how imbalances can lead to neuropathy.

Insulin Resistance: A Pathway to Neuropathy

Insulin resistance is a condition in which cells become less responsive to insulin. This can lead to elevated blood sugar levels, even when insulin levels are normal.

There are three stages of insulin resistance:

1. **Early warning signs:**

*   Cellular resistance to insulin: When cells become resistant to insulin, they do not take up glucose as efficiently from the bloodstream, leading to elevated post-meal blood sugar levels.
*   Elevated post-meal blood sugar levels: High blood sugar levels can damage nerves over time.

2. **Moderate insulin resistance:**

*   Impaired glucose tolerance: This condition is characterized by blood sugar levels that are higher than normal but not yet high enough to be diagnosed as diabetes.
*   Increased abdominal fat, metabolic syndrome, and neuropathy risk factors: Abdominal obesity and metabolic syndrome (high blood pressure, high blood sugar, excess body fat around the waist, and abnormal cholesterol levels) are both associated with insulin resistance and an increased risk of neuropathy.

3. Severe insulin resistance:

- Chronic high blood sugar levels: This can lead to several complications, including neuropathy.
- Beta-cell exhaustion and the inability to produce protective insulin: Over time, beta cells can become exhausted from overproducing insulin to compensate for insulin resistance. This can lead to decreased insulin production and worsening blood sugar control.

Lifestyle Tips to Improve Insulin Sensitivity

The good news is insulin resistance is a reversible condition. I often recommend the following lifestyle changes to my patients to help improve their insulin sensitivity:

- **Eat a healthy diet.** This means eating plenty of fruits, vegetables, and healthy protein sources (wild-caught fish, grass-fed beef and steak, free-range chicken, etc.). These foods are packed with essential vitamins, minerals, and antioxidants necessary for good health.

Limiting processed foods, sugary drinks, and unhealthy fats is also important.

When grocery shopping, focus on the store's perimeter, where fresh fruits, vegetables, whole grains, and lean protein sources will be found. Avoid the processed foods and sugary drinks in the center of the store.

- **Exercise regularly.** Exercise helps to improve insulin sensitivity and reduce blood sugar levels. Aim for at least 30 minutes of moderate-intensity exercise most days of the week. However, you may need to start slowly. Walking a block around your neighborhood is often a great way to start.

Find an activity that you enjoy and that fits into your schedule. Some easy ways to get more exercise include walking, hiking, biking, swimming, dancing, or taking a fitness class.

- **Lose weight if needed.** Excess weight can contribute to insulin resistance. Losing even a small amount of weight can make a big difference in improving insulin sensitivity.

At Optimal Performance Chiropractic, we can provide a healthy and sustainable weight loss plan based on your specific needs. Small changes, such as eating smaller portions, choosing more nutritious foods, or decreasing the hours of the day you eat, can make a big difference over time.

- **Get enough sleep.** When we don't get enough sleep, our bodies produce more of the stress hormone cortisol. Cortisol can promote insulin resistance. Aim for 7+ hours of QUALITY sleep each night. Quality can beat quantity when it comes to sleep.

Establish a regular sleep schedule and stick to it as much as possible, even on weekends. Create a relaxing bedtime routine that will help you wind down before bed. This should include eliminating blue light sources (computer, phone, and television screens) 60 minutes before bedtime.

Supplementing with magnesium and glycine before bed can also help calm your nervous system and result in higher-quality sleep.

- **Manage stress.** Stress can also promote insulin resistance. Find healthy ways to manage stress, such as exercise, yoga, or meditation. If you're feeling overwhelmed, talk to a mental health specialist.

In addition to the above lifestyle changes, people can do a few other things to improve their insulin sensitivity:

- **Take probiotics.** Probiotics are beneficial bacteria that live in the gut. Probiotics have been shown to improve insulin sensitivity and reduce blood sugar levels.
- **Take berberine.** Berberine is a plant compound that improves insulin sensitivity and reduces blood sugar levels.
- **Take cinnamon.** Cinnamon is another plant compound that has been shown to improve insulin sensitivity.

Making these lifestyle changes can take time and effort, but it's worth it for your health and well-being. By improving your insulin sensitivity, you can reduce your risk of developing neuropathy or other chronic diseases and live a longer, healthier life.

ACTION STEP: Insulin-glucagon balance is essential for maintaining healthy blood sugar levels. When this balance is disrupted, it can lead to many health problems, including neuropathy.

See if your blood sugar levels are higher than the normal range. If it's high, then we must get it under control to have a good chance of relieving neuropathy symptoms.

We will test fasting blood glucose and HbA1c. If you are interested in having your blood glucose level tested, scan the code below.

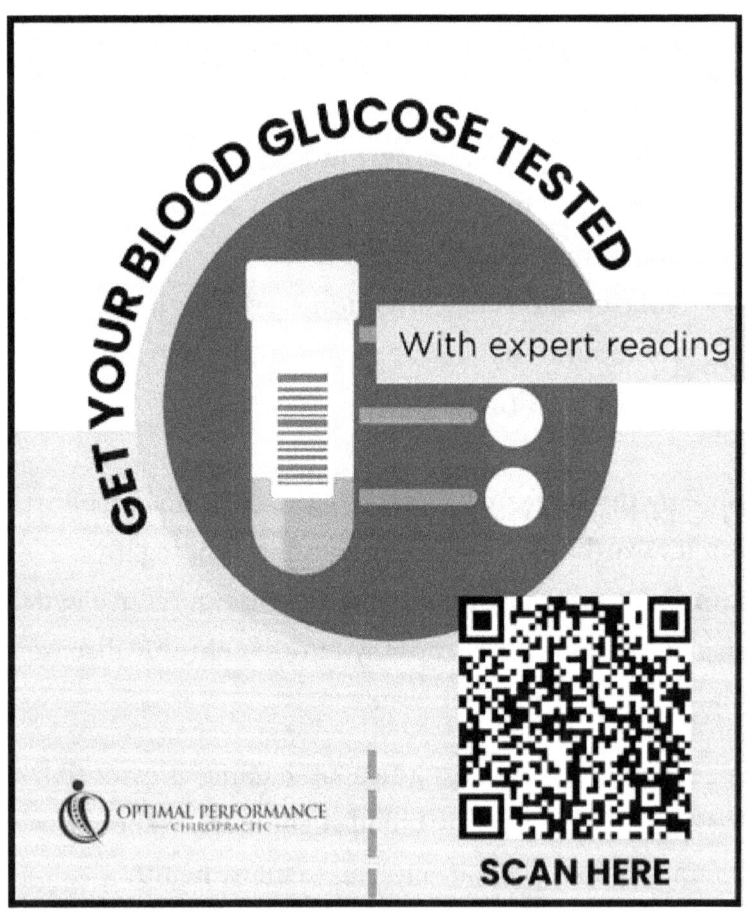

From Constant Pain to Restful Nights: Deborah's Neuropathy Recovery

"I was diagnosed with diabetes, and that's where my neuropathy started in my feet. I had horrible, horrible pain. I wasn't able to sleep at night, and nothing was helping. The medication my regular doctor gave me was just for the pain, but it really wasn't even helping that. And I was saddened to hear from her that it wasn't going to get better. It was only going to get worse. Eventually, I was looking at possible wheelchair. But within the first two weeks with Dr. Landry, it was a total change around. I had no more stabbing pains in my feet. I could sleep at night. It's just so much hope that I would wake up in the morning and go, wow. I actually slept all night. I wasn't up five, six times in such horrible pain just trying to walk it off and not interrupt my husband's sleep. I just want to keep moving forward with this and see what else it has to offer me."

** Every patient's journey is unique. This testimonial does not guarantee similar results for others.*

Unlock Your Path to Neuropathy Relief Now: Dial (951) 405-8868 to Speak With Us Today!

5

THE BODY'S OWN PHARMACY: HOLISTIC HEALING FOR NEUROPATHY

A few years ago, a patient named Sandra came to see me, defeated and disheartened. She was struggling with constant tingling and numbness in her hands, making even simple tasks like buttoning her blouse a challenge. She'd tried various medications, but the side effects were almost as unbearable as the neuropathy itself.

"Dr. Landry," she confessed, her voice tight with frustration, "I'm starting to think I'll never be able to enjoy cooking or knitting again. Is this just my life now?"

That's when we started to talk about the power of food as medicine. We worked together to create a personalized nutrition plan, focusing on whole, unprocessed foods and minimizing inflammatory triggers. Within a few weeks, Sandra noticed a significant difference. The tingling subsided, and the numbness lessened. By the end of her program, she was back to knitting beautiful scarves and whipping up delicious meals for her family. Of course, everyone's journey is unique, and individual results may vary. But Sandra's story beautifully illustrates how tapping into the body's innate healing potential – a potential often underestimated – can lead to remarkable results.

Neuropathy, with its diverse symptoms and complex nature, often leaves individuals seeking answers beyond solely medication. While medication can play a role, true healing often lies in unlocking the potential within your own body. In this chapter, we unveil a multifaceted approach that goes beyond symptom management, empowering you to actively participate in your journey towards well-being.

Fueling Resilience: A Dietary Approach to Preventing Neuropathy

The foods you eat play a vital role in your blood sugar levels. A low-glycemic, anti-inflammatory, and nutrient-dense diet is ideal for neuropathy prevention. Therefore, eat plenty of fruits, vegetables, and high-quality proteins and limit processed foods, sugary drinks, and unhealthy fats.

Fiber, healthy fats, and antioxidants are especially beneficial for nerve health. Fiber helps to regulate blood sugar levels, while healthy fats and antioxidants protect nerves from damage.

Here are some specific dietary tips for neuropathy prevention:

- Eat plenty of fruits, vegetables, and whole grains. They are packed with essential vitamins, minerals, and antioxidants necessary for good health. They are also low in calories and carbohydrates, which can help to keep blood sugar levels stable.
- Choose high-quality protein sources, such as wild-caught fish, free-range chicken, and grass-fed beef. High-quality protein sources are high in nutrients essential for nerve health, such as vitamin B12 and zinc.
- Limit trans fats. Trans fats can raise cholesterol levels and increase the risk of heart disease and stroke. They can also contribute to insulin resistance, which can lead to high blood sugar levels and neuropathy.
- Include healthy fats such as extra virgin olive oil, avocados, grass-fed butter, and nuts. Healthy fats can help to improve insulin

sensitivity and reduce inflammation. They can also protect nerves from damage.

- Avoid sugary drinks and processed foods. Sugary drinks and processed foods are often high in calories, carbohydrates, and unhealthy fats. They can also be low in essential nutrients. Consuming sugary drinks and processed foods can lead to high blood sugar levels and insulin resistance, which can increase the risk of neuropathy.

- Drink plenty of water. Staying hydrated is vital for overall health and well-being. It is also essential for nerve health. When we are dehydrated, our blood sugar levels can rise. This can damage nerves and increase the risk of neuropathy.

By following these dietary tips, you can help to improve your blood sugar control and protect your nerves from damage.

ACTION STEP: Put mineral salt in your drinking water to stay properly hydrated.

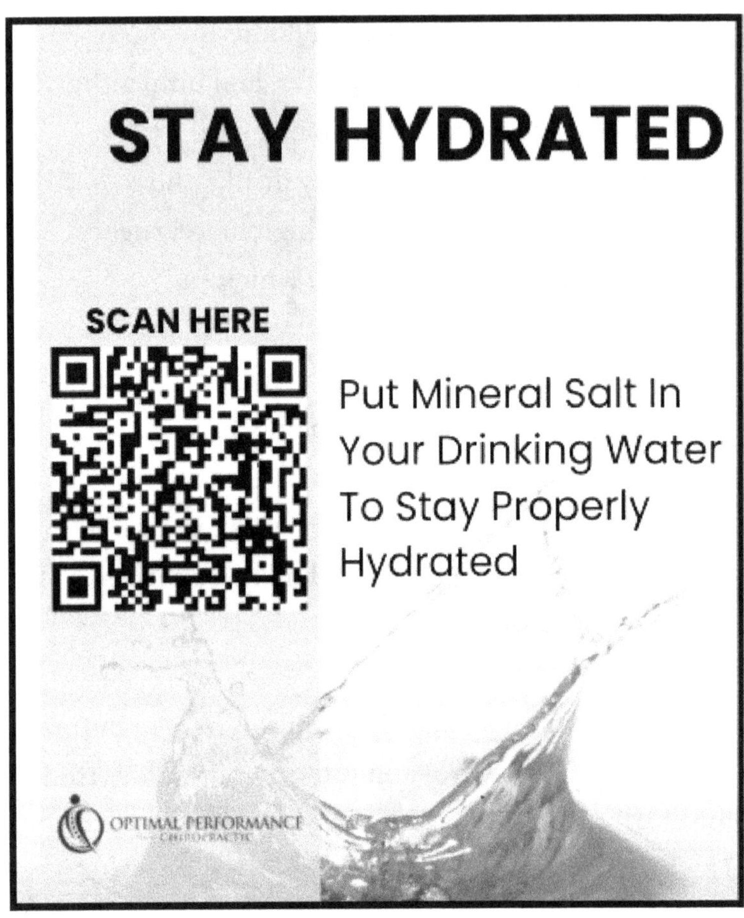

Diet Transformations and Their Impact

Diet transformations can profoundly impact nerve health. When we switch to a healthy diet full of nutrient-rich foods, we can see improvements in nerve function and reduce our risk of developing neuropathy and many other diseases.

Here are some of the benefits of a diet transformation for nerve health:

- **Reduced inflammation:** Inflammation is a major contributor to nerve damage. A healthy diet can help to reduce inflammation throughout the body, including the nervous system.
- **Improved blood sugar control:** High blood sugar levels can damage nerves over time, acting like a chronic poison. When blood sugar stays elevated, it coats the delicate nerves like syrup, interfering with their ability to send signals properly. This can lead to tingling, numbness, and eventually, even complete loss of nerve function. A healthy diet can help regulate blood sugar and prevent this nerve damage.
- **Increased nutrient intake:** Nerves need various nutrients to function properly. A healthy diet can help ensure we get the nutrients we need for nerve health, such as B vitamins, magnesium, and omega-3 fatty acids.

When making a diet transformation, remember to make gradual changes. Don't try to change your entire diet overnight. Start with a few small changes and build from there. Let me share a few healthy meal plans and recipes to get you started.

Meal Plans and Recipes for Nerve Health

Here is a sample meal plan for a day of eating for nerve health:

Breakfast:

- Hard-boiled eggs
- Whole-wheat toast with avocado

Lunch:

- Salad with grilled chicken or fish OR
- Quinoa bowl with black beans, roasted vegetables, and avocado

Dinner:

- Salmon with roasted vegetables and brown rice OR
- Chicken stir-fry with brown rice or quinoa
- Lentil soup

Snacks:

- Fruits and vegetables
- Nuts and seeds
- Yogurt with berries and nuts

Recipes

Salad with Grilled Chicken or Fish

Ingredients:

- Mixed greens
- Grilled chicken or fish
- Tomatoes
- Cucumbers
- Onions
- Avocado
- Olive oil
- Vinegar
- Salt and pepper

Instructions:

1. Toss together the greens, grilled chicken or fish, tomatoes, cucumbers, onions, and avocado.

2. Drizzle with olive oil and vinegar.
3. Season with salt and pepper to taste.
4. Serve and enjoy!

Salmon with Roasted Vegetables and Brown Rice

Ingredients:

- 1 salmon filet
- 1 tablespoon olive oil
- 1/2 teaspoon salt
- 1/4 teaspoon black pepper
- 1 cup roasted vegetables (such as broccoli, Brussels sprouts, and carrots)
- 1 cup cooked brown rice

Instructions:

1. Preheat the oven to 400 degrees Fahrenheit.
2. Place the salmon filet on a baking sheet.
3. Drizzle with olive oil and season with salt and pepper.
4. Bake for 12-15 minutes, or until the salmon is cooked through.
5. Serve with roasted vegetables and brown rice.

Chicken Stir-Fry with Brown Rice or Quinoa

Ingredients:

- 1 pound boneless, skinless chicken breasts, cut into bite-sized pieces
- 1 tablespoon olive oil
- 1/2 onion, chopped
- 2 cloves garlic, minced
- 1 bell pepper, sliced
- 1 cup broccoli florets
- 1/2 cup carrots, sliced
- 1/4 cup soy sauce
- 1/4 cup rice vinegar
- 1 tablespoon cornstarch
- 1 tablespoon water
- Salt and pepper to taste
- 1 cup cooked brown rice or quinoa

Instructions:

1. Heat the olive oil in a large skillet over medium heat.
2. Add the chicken and cook until browned on all sides.
3. Add the onion, garlic, bell pepper, and broccoli.

4. Cook until the vegetables are tender.
5. In a small bowl, whisk together the soy sauce, rice vinegar, cornstarch, and water.
6. Add the sauce to the skillet and cook until thickened.
7. Season with salt and pepper to taste.
8. Serve over cooked brown rice or quinoa.

Lentil Soup

Ingredients:

- 1 cup lentils
- 2 cups vegetable broth
- 1 onion, chopped
- 2 carrots, chopped
- 2 celery stalks, chopped
- 1 teaspoon garlic powder
- 1/2 teaspoon dried thyme
- 1/4 teaspoon black pepper
- 1/4 teaspoon salt

Instructions:

1. Rinse the lentils in a fine-mesh strainer.
2. Place the lentils, vegetable broth, onion, carrots, celery, garlic powder, thyme, pepper, and salt in a slow cooker.

3. Cook on low for 6-8 hours, or until the lentils are tender.

4. Serve warm and enjoy!

These are just a few examples of healthy and delicious meals and snacks that are good for nerve health. Following these tips can help protect your nerves and reduce your risk of developing neuropathy.

Unleashing Movement's Healing Potential: Physical Therapy and Exercise in Neuropathy Management

Living with neuropathy often leads to limitations in movement, contributing to pain and reducing quality of life. But did you know that movement itself can be a powerful tool in managing your condition? Physical therapy and exercise, carefully tailored to your needs, can unlock a secret weapon in your fight against neuropathy – your own body's healing potential.

Defining the Power of Movement

Physical therapy and exercise offer a multi-pronged approach to addressing neuropathy:

- **Improving nerve function:** Specific exercises stimulate nerve pathways, promoting regeneration and reducing pain signals.

- **Enhancing muscle strength and flexibility:** This helps maintain balance, prevent falls, and reduce pain due to muscle imbalances.
- **Boosting circulation:** Increased blood flow nourishes nerves and delivers essential nutrients for healing.
- **Promoting overall well-being:** Exercise releases endorphins, natural mood enhancers that combat depression and anxiety often associated with chronic pain.

Examples of Effective Programs

- **Balance and gait training:** Regaining confident mobility reduces fall risk and improves daily activities.
- **Aerobic exercise:** Walking, swimming, or cycling improves cardiovascular health and circulation, promoting nerve health.
- **Strength training:** Targeted exercises build muscle strength and support, alleviating pain and improving function.
- **Stretching and flexibility exercises:** Improving flexibility reduces stiffness and muscle tightness, contributing to pain relief.

While physical therapy and exercise programs may incur initial costs, consider them an investment in your long-term health and well-being. The benefits often outweigh the cost:

- **Reduced pain and improved quality of life:** Less reliance on pain medication, increased independence, and a more active lifestyle.
- **Prevention of complications:** Maintaining strength and balance reduces fall risk and other potential complications.
- **Improved mental well-being:** Exercise combats depression and anxiety, boosting overall well-being.

Empowering Actions

1. **Talk to your doctor** and discuss your interest in physical therapy and exercise. We can recommend a program tailored to your specific needs and limitations.
2. **Seek a qualified therapist** who prioritizes personalized care plans and offers a variety of treatments tailored to your unique needs and goals. The team at Optimal Performance Chiropractic embraces this individualized

approach, working collaboratively with you to develop a plan that aligns with your specific health aspirations.

3. **Start gradually** with low-impact exercises and gradually increase intensity and duration as your fitness improves.

4. **Consistency is key:** Regular exercise is crucial for long-term benefits. Aim for at least 30 minutes of moderate-intensity exercise most days of the week.

5. **Listen to your body:** Don't push yourself beyond your limits; take rest days when needed. Communicate any pain or discomfort to your therapist.

Remember, unlocking the secrets of movement requires taking the first step. Incorporating physical therapy and exercise into your neuropathy management plan can empower your body to heal, regain strength, and reclaim your active life.

Quieting the Inner Storm: How Stress Management Benefits Neuropathy

Living with neuropathy often feels like a constant battle against pain, but did you know that another, less obvious foe lurks in the shadows – stress? Chronic stress can significantly worsen your symptoms, creating a vicious cycle of discomfort and anxiety.

But there's good news! By incorporating effective stress management techniques into your neuropathy management plan, you can unlock a powerful tool for reducing pain and reclaiming your well-being.

Understanding the Stress-Neuropathy Connection

Stress triggers the release of hormones like cortisol, which, in excess, can damage nerve cells and exacerbate inflammation, both key players in neuropathy. Additionally, stress can:

- **Increase pain perception:** When stressed, your body becomes more sensitive to pain signals, making existing neuropathy symptoms feel worse.
- **Disrupt sleep:** Poor sleep quality further fuels stress and inflammation, hindering nerve healing and recovery.
- **Weaken the immune system:** Chronic stress weakens your body's defenses, making you more susceptible to infections, which can worsen neuropathy symptoms.

Examples of Stress Management Techniques

Fortunately, various techniques can help quiet the inner storm and promote healing:

- **Mindfulness and meditation:** These practices train your mind to focus on the present moment, reducing anxious thoughts and calming the nervous system.
- **Yoga and deep breathing:** Yoga combines physical postures, breathing exercises, and meditation, promoting relaxation and stress reduction.
- **Progressive muscle relaxation:** This technique involves systematically tensing and releasing different muscle groups, promoting physical and mental relaxation.
- **Biofeedback:** This technique uses technology to help you become aware of your body's stress response and learn to control it.
- **Spending time in nature:** Immersing yourself in nature has proven stress-reducing effects, promoting both physical and mental well-being.

While some stress management techniques require no financial investment, others, like therapy or biofeedback, may incur costs. However, consider these benefits:

- **Reduced pain and improved quality of life:** Less stress means less pain and a calmer, more enjoyable life.
- **Improved sleep:** Better sleep promotes healing and boosts overall well-being.
- **Enhanced emotional well-being:** Managing stress reduces anxiety and depression, often associated with chronic pain.

Empowering Actions

1. **Identify your stress triggers.** What situations or thoughts cause you stress? Awareness is the first step in managing it.
2. **Explore different techniques.** Experiment with various methods to find what resonates with you.
3. **Start small and be consistent.** Begin with short practice sessions and gradually increase as you get comfortable.
4. **Seek professional guidance.** Consider therapy or workshops for deeper stress management strategies.

5. **Find a support system.** Connect with friends, family, or support groups for encouragement and shared experiences.

Remember, stress management is not a one-time fix; it's an ongoing journey. By incorporating these techniques into your daily life, you can quiet the inner storm of stress and empower your body to heal from neuropathy. Take control of your well-being, one calming breath at a time.

Beyond the Usual Suspects: Unveiling Integrative Medicine for Neuropathy Relief

Neuropathy's complex nature often demands a multifaceted approach. While conventional medicine plays a crucial role, integrative medicine offers a unique perspective, weaving together various complementary therapies to support your body's natural healing mechanisms.

In this section, we unveil the potential of this holistic approach, empowering you to explore its benefits and make informed decisions for your well-being.

Defining Integrative Medicine

Integrative medicine goes beyond solely treating symptoms. It addresses the root causes of neuropathy while considering your whole being – physical, emotional, and spiritual. This holistic approach often combines conventional therapies with complementary and alternative therapies, creating a personalized plan tailored to your unique needs.

Examples of Integrative Approaches

- **Chiropractic care:** Chiropractic adjustments aim to improve spinal alignment and function, potentially reducing nerve compression and alleviating pain associated with neuropathy.
- **Acupuncture:** This ancient practice involves inserting thin needles at specific points to stimulate the nervous system and promote healing. It may help reduce pain, improve sleep, and manage stress.
- **Massage therapy:** Gentle massage techniques can improve circulation, reduce muscle tension, and promote relaxation, potentially alleviating pain and improving sleep quality.
- **Herbal remedies:** Certain herbs, like turmeric and ginger, possess anti-inflammatory properties that may offer pain relief and support nerve health. It is crucial to consult with a qualified healthcare professional before using any herbal remedies.

- **Mind-body therapies:** Techniques like meditation and yoga can effectively manage stress, improve sleep, and promote overall well-being, indirectly contributing to neuropathy management.

Integrative medicine therapies can vary in cost depending on the specific approach and practitioner. While some may incur additional expenses, consider the potential benefits:

- **Reduced pain and improved quality of life:** A holistic approach can address various aspects influencing neuropathy, potentially leading to significant pain relief and improved overall well-being.
- **Addressing root causes:** Integrative medicine may offer long-term solutions beyond symptom management by exploring underlying factors like stress or inflammation.
- **Empowering your body:** Engaging in complementary therapies can empower you to actively participate in your healing journey, fostering a sense of control and well-being.

Taking Action

1. **Talk to your doctor.** Discuss your interest in integrative medicine and explore options suitable for your specific condition.
2. **Seek qualified practitioners.** Ensure chosen practitioners are licensed and have experience treating neuropathy with their chosen modality.
3. **Start cautiously.** Begin with a single therapy and gradually incorporate others as you feel comfortable.
4. **Communicate openly.** Keep your doctor informed about any complementary therapies you use to ensure safe and coordinated care.
5. **Be patient and persistent.** Integrative medicine often requires time and commitment to see results. Trust the process and celebrate even small improvements.

Remember, integrative medicine is not a replacement for conventional treatment but rather a valuable complement. By exploring its potential, including chiropractic care, you can unlock a new dimension of healing and empower your body to manage neuropathy holistically and sustainably. Let your journey begin with an open mind and a willingness to explore the possibilities!

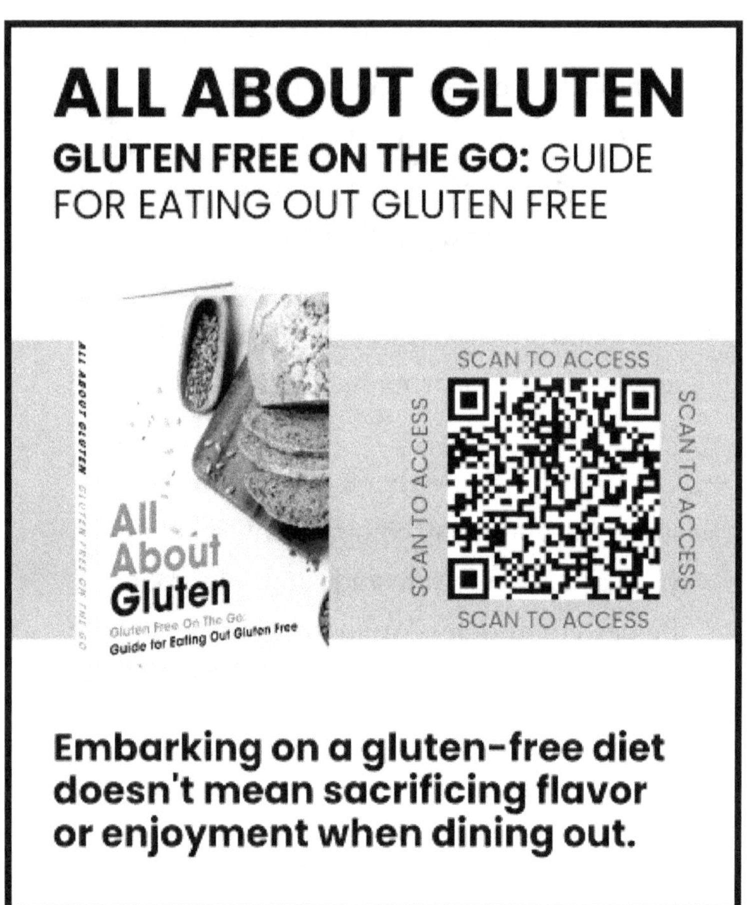

Unlock Your Path to Neuropathy Relief Now: Dial (951) 405-8868 to Speak With Us Today!

6

———

QUICK FIXES & FALSE HOPE: WHY SOME TREATMENTS DON'T WORK

Living with neuropathy, the persistent pain and numbness that steals vitality, often leads individuals to desperately seek immediate relief. Home remedies, readily available supplements, and promises of miracle cures whisper hope, but do they deliver lasting results?

In this chapter, we embark on a journey of truth-seeking, dissecting the allure and limitations of common quick fixes. From exploring the unregulated world of home remedies to examining the claims behind popular supplements, we'll unveil why these approaches often fall short.

But this isn't just about exposing shortcomings; it's about empowering you with knowledge and guiding you towards a more effective path. By understanding the pitfalls and limitations of quick fixes, you'll be better equipped to embrace a comprehensive, evidence-based approach that paves the way for a brighter future – a future beyond neuropathy's shadows.

Why Home Remedies Fall Flat

When I first learned about the power and importance of Vitamin D for health and performance, I immediately started supplementing with it. This was especially important for me through the winter months as sunshine is minimal, so the body is not producing its own vitamin D at a proper level.

Unfortunately, after a couple of months of supplementation, I did not notice any positive results. That is when I dug deeper into the science and realized that all fat-soluble vitamins work together in harmony, and supplementing only one of them does not give adequate results.

Vitamins D, A, K, & E should be taken together to get optimal results for your physiology. What I learned was that everything in the human body works together synergistically, and using one approach by itself is nowhere near as effective. This is the problem we see time and again with home remedies for neuropathy.

Home remedies for neuropathy are often hailed as quick fixes. From essential oils to over-the-counter creams, these treatments are frequently endorsed in the court of public opinion, social media forums, or anecdotal evidence.

While they may promise quick relief, it's crucial to separate the wheat from the chaff and understand why these methods generally fall short of providing a lasting solution to neuropathy.

We hear so many stories of people who have tried home remedies and failed. Like John, a 60-year-old man who was desperate to find relief from his neuropathy. He tried every home remedy he came across - essential oils, over-the-counter creams, and even some obscure vitamins recommended in an online advertisement.

Each new remedy brought a glimmer of hope, but the relief was always fleeting. The tingling and numbness in his feet persisted, leaving him frustrated and discouraged. It was only when he sought professional help that he began to see real progress in managing his symptoms.

Other countless individuals grasp at straws, hoping the next 'miracle cure' they read about online will be the answer to their painful symptoms. From creams that promise to 'burn away' pain to soaking feet in tonic water, people have gone to great lengths, only to find these methods offer, at best, temporary relief.

While home remedies may seem like a tempting option for quick relief, the costs of pursuing them can be significant, both financially and physically. Time is a valuable resource, and spending hours researching and applying home remedies can quickly add up. Additionally, the cost of these treatments can accumulate, especially if you are trying multiple remedies at once.

Even more concerning is the potential danger of home remedies. Using improper concentrations or mixing different solutions can lead to adverse reactions, such as skin irritation, inflammation, and even nerve damage.

Perform a cost-benefit analysis before trying any home remedy. Weigh the financial and health-related costs against the potential benefits. If the financial and health-related costs of the home remedy outweigh the potential benefits, it is best to avoid it. Instead, visit optimalperformancechiropractic.com and request an appointment to learn more effective and safe treatment options.

Remember, your health is your most important asset. Don't put it at risk by trying unproven or unsafe home remedies.

The Allure and Failings of Supplements

Supplements are big business. In the United States, people spend billions of dollars annually on supplements, including vitamins, minerals, herbs, and other botanicals. The appeal of supplements is understandable. They promise to improve our health, boost our energy, and help us lose weight. But the reality is that many supplements are ineffective and even dangerous.

There are several reasons why supplements often fail to live up to their claims. First, the supplement industry is largely unregulated. This means that manufacturers can make bold claims about their products without having to back them up with scientific evidence.

The most common problem with this is companies advertising a "studied" ingredient in their supplement, only to find out that the study was done with a much higher dosage than they provide in their supplement. Second, many supplements are not well-studied, so we don't know how safe or effective they are. Third, supplements can interact with other medications and supplements, causing unexpected side effects.

Our industry has seen firsthand the harm that supplements can cause. We've seen people who spent thousands of dollars on supplements that were marketed to help relieve neuropathy. Unfortunately, none of those supplements worked, and some of them even made symptoms worse. Other people have even developed liver damage from taking a supplement that was marketed to improve blood sugar control.

A prime example of this is vitamin B6. The synthetic version (pyridoxine) that is found in many supplements is not biocompatible and can cause harm to the human body, including causing neuropathy symptoms. However, the naturally occurring form of vitamin B6 (Pyridoxal-5-Phosphate) can actually IMPROVE neuropathy symptoms.

While more research needs to be done on the efficacy of supplements in treating neuropathy, here are proven supplements and vitamins that can help:

- L-Citrulline, a nitric oxide precursor
- L-Glutathione, an antioxidant produced by the liver and nerve cells
- Vitamin B-12, to help with nerve function
- Acetyl-L-carnitine, an antioxidant
- Alpha-lipoic acid, an antioxidant that can help treat neuropathy caused by diabetes
- Amarasate, a hops plant extract. This helps reduce cravings for sugar by up to 30%.

If you are considering taking supplements, it's essential to do your research and talk to your doctor. Choose supplements from reputable manufacturers and avoid supplements that make unrealistic claims. It's also important to be aware of the potential side effects and interactions of supplements.

Why Quick Fixes Fail on the Neuropathy Journey

The lure of a "quick fix" can be tempting, especially when facing the challenges of neuropathy. However, the reality is that lasting solutions rarely reside in instant cures or miracle products. Let's have a look at the fallacy of quick fixes and empower you to embrace sustainable approaches for effective neuropathy management.

The Allure and the Illusion

The desire for an immediate solution is understandable. Pain, discomfort, and limitations can fuel a yearning for a magic bullet that swiftly erases neuropathy and its impact. Unfortunately, quick fixes often:

- **Lack of scientific backing:** They rarely have robust evidence supporting their claims and often rely on anecdotes or testimonials rather than rigorous research.

- **Promise unrealistic results:** They often oversimplify the complex nature of neuropathy, offering unrealistic expectations of complete cures or instant pain relief.
- **Address symptoms, not the root cause:** They might temporarily mask symptoms but fail to address the underlying mechanisms driving nerve damage, leading to recurring issues.
- **Pose potential risks:** Some quick fixes can have harmful side effects or interact with medications, jeopardizing your overall well-being.

Embracing the Sustainable Path

While a magical solution might seem appealing, the reality is that lasting progress often requires a multifaceted and sustainable approach. This might involve:

- **Early diagnosis and intervention:** Seeking professional help early allows for identifying the root cause and implementing effective treatment strategies before further damage occurs.

- **Holistic approach:** This encompasses various evidence-based practices and lifestyle modifications working in harmony to address the physical, emotional, and even spiritual aspects of neuropathy. This could include:
  - Mind-body practices: Techniques like meditation and yoga can help manage pain, improve sleep, and reduce anxiety associated with neuropathy.
  - Dietary changes: Focusing on anti-inflammatory and nutrient-rich foods can support nerve health and overall well-being.
  - Exercising regularly: Appropriate physical activity helps improve circulation, manage pain, and maintain mobility.
  - Stress management: Techniques like deep breathing and relaxation exercises can help reduce stress, a known contributor to neuropathy symptoms.
  - Supplements: When recommended by a healthcare professional, specific supplements can support nerve health based on individual needs.

Forget the fairytale: there's no magic cure for neuropathy. Lasting progress requires dedication and commitment to a multifaceted approach. Yes, it takes time and effort, but the rewards are worth it.

Instead of chasing overnight miracles, celebrate every step forward, no matter how small. Each sustainable change you integrate into your routine, whether it's a mindful meditation practice, a nutritious meal, or a gentle exercise session, adds another brick to the foundation of your long-term nerve health.

Remember, patience is key. Dedication to evidence-based strategies, like those offered by your healthcare professional, unlocks the door to lasting solutions for managing neuropathy. Embrace the journey, celebrate your progress, and never lose sight of the possibility for improvement.

All That Glitters Isn't Gold: Real Stories Expose the Pitfalls of Quick Fixes

The allure of a "quick fix" for neuropathy can be strong, especially when faced with pain, discomfort, and limitations. But as tempting as these promises may seem, countless individuals have learned the hard way that they often fall short, leading to disappointment and frustration. Let's look at some real stories of failed quick fixes, exposing their pitfalls and empowering you to make informed choices on your journey toward effective neuropathy management.

The Bioenergetic Bluff

Mark, a retired carpenter with carpal tunnel syndrome, invested in a bioenergetic bracelet advertised to "rebalance his energy" and alleviate his pain. Despite wearing it constantly and following the specific activation rituals, he experienced no improvement and later learned from his doctor that such bracelets lacked any scientific basis for pain relief.

The Detox Disaster

Lisa, a young woman diagnosed with autoimmune neuropathy, attempted a strict homemade detox regimen based on online recommendations. While initially enthusiastic, the restrictive diet and intense cleanses led to nutrient deficiencies, worsening fatigue, and increased anxiety. This experience emphasized the importance of consulting healthcare professionals before embarking on any drastic dietary changes.

A Musician's Brush with Unregulated Supplements

David, a musician with peripheral neuropathy, opted for an herbal remedy promoted online as a "natural cure" due to concerns about potential side effects from conventional medications. Unfortunately, the unregulated nature of the supplement led to unknown interactions with his current medications, causing adverse reactions and requiring medical intervention.

This story highlights the importance of consulting healthcare professionals before utilizing unregulated supplements.

These stories highlight the common pitfalls of quick fixes:

- **False promises and unrealistic expectations:** Quick fixes often oversimplify complex conditions like neuropathy, leading to disappointment when results don't match the hype.
- **Lack of scientific evidence:** Many quick fixes rely on anecdotal claims and lack robust research to support their effectiveness or safety.
- **Potential for harm:** Some quick fixes can have adverse side effects or interact with medications, jeopardizing your overall well-being.
- **Unsustainable solutions:** They rarely address the underlying causes of neuropathy, leading to recurring issues and dependence on the product.

Empowering Yourself for Lasting Progress

Instead of chasing quick fixes, focus on sustainable approaches proven to manage neuropathy effectively:

- **Seek professional diagnosis and guidance:** Early intervention by qualified healthcare professionals allows for identifying the root cause and implementing evidence-based treatment plans.

- **Embrace a holistic approach:** This involves a combination of strategies like medication, physical therapy, lifestyle modifications, and mind-body practices, addressing the physical, emotional, and even spiritual aspects of neuropathy.

- **Prioritize healthy habits:** Regular exercise, a balanced diet, stress management, and adequate sleep can significantly improve nerve health and overall well-being.

- **Be patient and consistent:** Lasting progress takes time and dedication. Celebrate small improvements and focus on building sustainable habits for long-term success.

By understanding the limitations of quick fixes and prioritizing evidence-based approaches, you can empower yourself to manage neuropathy and reclaim your well-being effectively.

The Importance of Patient Education

Neuropathy can feel like you're lost at sea, navigating through choppy waters with no compass or map in sight. But knowledge is your lighthouse, casting a beacon of hope on the path toward reclaiming your life. It's more than just facts and figures; it's about understanding your condition inside and out, empowering you to take the helm of your health journey.

I've seen countless individuals transform their lives simply by learning about neuropathy. They become captains of their own ships, steering confidently through stormy seas. The power of knowledge is truly remarkable; it gives you the tools to make informed decisions, advocate for yourself, and ultimately, find your way back to calmer waters.

Knowing what's going on with your body is the first step towards taking control of your health. It allows you to collaborate with healthcare professionals, ask the right questions, and be an active part of your treatment. You're not just a bystander anymore, but a key player in your journey back to feeling your best. YOU are the captain of this ship.

Nowadays, information is everywhere. Everything is just a click away. But sifting through the internet can be like getting lost in a maze of data. It's like having a library card but no librarian to guide you to the correct stuff. That's why reliable sources and trusted healthcare providers are so important.

Not all information is created equal. You might stumble across some tempting "miracle cures" while researching neuropathy, but remember, some of these might be too good to be true. This flood of information can be confusing and frustrating, especially when it comes to a complicated condition like neuropathy.

Consider the story of John, which we discussed earlier in this chapter. Desperate to find relief, John tried countless home remedies, but the results were always fleeting. Had he been properly educated about neuropathy, he could have avoided unnecessary expense and disappointment. Misinformation and anecdotal evidence can lead individuals down a path that fails to provide relief and can be financially costly and potentially harmful.

Navigating the complexities of healthcare information can feel overwhelming. It's crucial to find a team you trust, who prioritize a collaborative, patient-centered approach. At Optimal Performance Chiropractic, we believe in empowering our patients through education and offering individualized care plans that are grounded in evidence-based practices. We're dedicated to helping you make informed choices for your health, tailoring our approach to your unique needs and goals, and ensuring you feel confident in your path toward better well-being.

When you are well-informed and collaborate with holistic healthcare professionals, you can confidently pursue treatments that have a scientific basis and a higher likelihood of success. You avoid the pitfalls of unproven methods, save valuable time, and protect your most important asset—your health.

ACTION STEP: Scan the code below to download our 25 Anti-Inflammatory Recipes Guide.

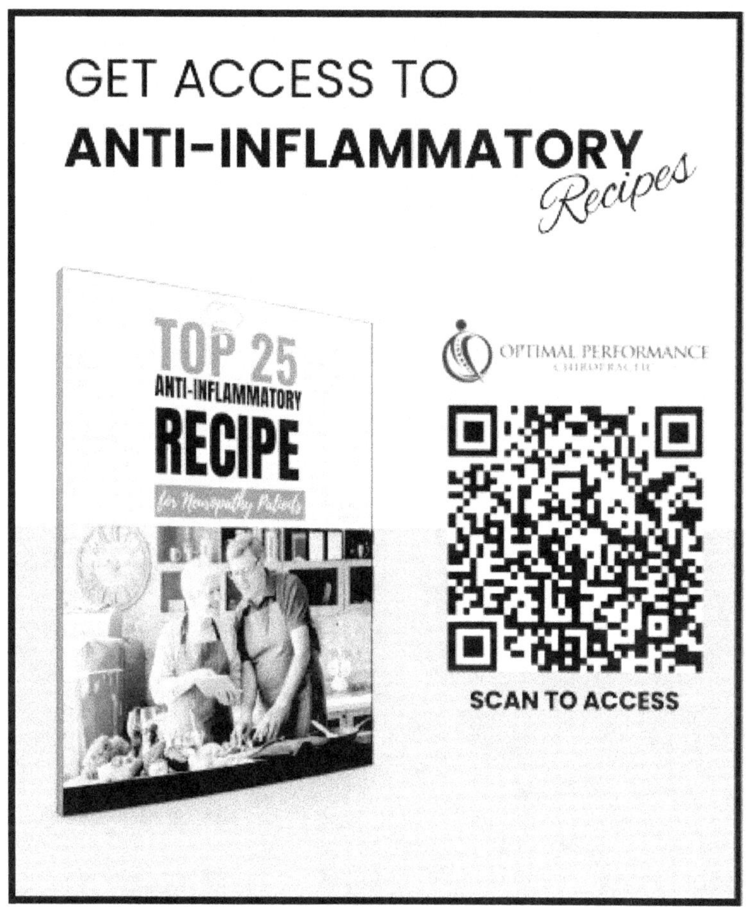

Ricky: "After COVID, RESTORE Was My Neuropathy Lifeline"

Optimal Performance Chiropractic is one of the most professional and competent I have encountered since 2020, when I was medically retired as a 1st Responder.

The state-of-the-art clinical procedures and home care treatments, coupled with nutritional supplements, have yielded the best results in dealing with the inflammation, neuropathy, and loss of mobility that has plagued me since my work-related exposure to COVID-19 and my subsequent hospitalization in the ICU. Years later, RESTORE is one of the few programs that have helped me regain my quality of life.

Individual outcomes may differ.

Unlock Your Path to Neuropathy Relief Now: Dial (951) 405-8868 to Speak With Us Today!

7

BREAKING THE MYTHS: TRUTH & HOPE FOR NEUROPATHY

I remember a patient, let's call him Mark, who came to me convinced his neuropathy was a life sentence. He'd been told by another doctor that there was nothing more to be done, that he should just accept his fate of increasing pain and limitations.

"Dr. Landry," he said, his voice thick with resignation, "I guess I'm just going to have to learn to live with this. It's only going to get worse, right?"

That statement, so steeped in despair, ignited a fire in me. I knew we had to shatter those limiting beliefs. Over the next few weeks, we worked together, addressing not only the physical aspects of his neuropathy but also the emotional and mental toll it had taken. We explored lifestyle changes, natural therapies, and empowered him with knowledge about his condition.

Slowly, but surely, Mark started to see progress. The pain lessened, his mobility improved, and most importantly, a flicker of hope rekindled in his eyes. He realized he wasn't powerless against his neuropathy, that there was a path forward, even if it wasn't the instant cure he'd initially hoped for. While each person's journey is unique and individual results may vary, Mark's transformation demonstrated the profound power of dispelling myths and embracing a proactive, informed approach to managing neuropathy.

Neuropathy casts a long shadow, often shrouded in misinformation and misconceptions. These myths can delay diagnosis, impede treatment, and fuel fear, leaving you feeling powerless in the face of this condition. But what if you could shatter these myths, revealing a path to empowered management and a brighter future?

Let's shatter some of these common myths surrounding neuropathy.

There is No Cure for Neuropathy

I've encountered this misconception many times, and it's crucial to address it. It's important to understand that neuropathy is a complex condition with various causes and manifestations. It's not a one-size-fits-all situation. The treatment and prognosis can vary greatly depending on the individual's health status, the type of neuropathy, and its underlying cause.

Now, let's talk about the myth that there's no cure for neuropathy. It's true that in some cases, especially when the damage to the nerves is severe or the cause is irreversible, complete recovery might not be possible. However, this doesn't mean that all hope is lost or that the condition can't be managed effectively.

In many cases, if the underlying cause of the neuropathy can be identified and treated, the nerves can heal, and the symptoms can be relieved. For instance, if the neuropathy is due to vitamin B12 deficiency, replenishing the body's B12 levels can often lead to significant improvement or even complete resolution of the symptoms.

Even in cases where the neuropathy is more chronic, and the nerve damage is extensive, there are still treatment options available, like our RESTORE program, that can help manage the symptoms and improve your quality of life. We use a non-invasive, holistic approach that includes the latest technology to help regenerate your nerves, chiropractic care to improve mobility and dietary modifications.

So, while it's true that there's currently no 'magic bullet' that can cure all forms of neuropathy, it's absolutely false to say that there's no hope or no treatment options available. Many RESTORE neuropathy patients are leading a normal and fulfilling life with the RESTORE healing framework.

Remember, it's always important to seek professional medical advice if you're experiencing symptoms of neuropathy. Early intervention is key to preventing further nerve damage and managing the condition effectively. Don't let myths and misconceptions stand in the way of getting the help you need. Your health is too important to leave to chance.

Enduring Pain Leads to Recovery

One of the most dangerous myths surrounding neuropathy is the belief that suffering through pain will somehow lead to recovery. It's an old-school approach echoing the "no pain, no gain" mentality, often leaving patients feeling that their struggle is a necessary rite of passage toward healing. The reality is far from this; ignoring the signs your body gives you can lead to aggravated symptoms and possibly irreversible damage.

We've seen it time and time again: the people with neuropathy who have bought into this myth are convinced that enduring the discomfort is the path to recovery. They soldier on for many months. The pain or numbness and tingling in their hands and feet became their constant companion, reminding them of their supposed resilience.

As time passed, their condition deteriorated. Simple tasks turned into Herculean efforts, but they pressed on, convinced they were on the right track. By the time they sought professional help, the damage had become extensive. Their neuropathy had progressed to a severe stage, leaving their mobility compromised and their quality of life severely diminished.

It's a harsh awakening for them. Believing you must suffer to recover can lead to grim scenarios. Patients delay seeking help, leading to worse symptoms, more pain, and even the loss of mobility. Instead of healing, this mindset often traps individuals in a vicious cycle of escalating agony.

And this harmful belief costs more than you can imagine. What starts as mild symptoms can escalate into chronic conditions or even irreversible damage because of this "suffer to get better" myth. This includes the loss of nerve function, muscle mass, and even the ability to walk.

The physical and emotional toll of this belief system is immense. The constant pain, the loss of mobility, and the degradation of quality of life are just the tip of the iceberg. The psychological impact of enduring constant pain, believing it to be a path to recovery, can lead to feelings of fatigue, depression, and anxiety.

Ignoring these signals that something is wrong and choosing to endure the pain can lead to irreversible damage. It's time to debunk this myth and spread awareness about the importance of seeking professional help when dealing with neuropathy. Early intervention can prevent the progression of the disease and improve the quality of life for those suffering from this condition.

Remember, enduring pain does not lead to recovery. It's not a sign of resilience but a warning sign that should not be ignored. Seek help, listen to your body, and take the necessary steps toward recovery. Don't let the myth of suffering through pain trap you in a cycle of escalating agony. Your health and well-being are too important to risk on a false belief.

Now, let's shift gears and talk about the practical steps you can take to navigate the path of neuropathy recovery. It's crucial to replace this outdated myth with informed, data-driven actions. This approach not only prevents potentially irreversible damage but sets you on the course toward regaining control and living pain-free. Here's how you can do it:

1. **Seek Early Intervention:** Remember, the sooner you address neuropathy, the better the chances of positive outcomes. Don't hold off until it reaches a crisis point.

2. **Data-Driven Analysis:** It's all about understanding the specifics of your condition. Medical assessments and tests can provide valuable insights into the severity of your neuropathy. This data is a crucial compass on your journey to recovery.

3. **Seek Specialized Support:** Finding the right healthcare provider is crucial when dealing with complex conditions. Look for a team experienced in non-surgical approaches to managing neuropathy, and who focus on addressing its underlying causes. The team at Optimal Performance Chiropractic prioritizes a holistic and comprehensive approach to your health and well-being.

4. **Holistic Care:** Look for therapies that go beyond just alleviating symptoms. Aim for treatments that target the root cause of your neuropathy. This holistic approach can lead to more sustained relief and long-term improvements in your quality of life.

Taking these steps is like building a solid foundation for your journey towards pain-free living. It's a roadmap that prioritizes early action, data-backed decisions, professional guidance, and comprehensive care. Remember, you've got this!

The Mirage of the Miracle Cure

In a world obsessed with quick fixes, the notion that a single pill can be the magic bullet for neuropathy is tempting but misleading. Many fall into this trap, thinking that pharmaceuticals will provide a comprehensive solution.

But the reality is a majority of people who rely solely on medications for neuropathy find that they only provide temporary relief. The symptoms return once the medication wears off, and in some cases, the medication can even cause side effects that worsen the condition.

One typical example is the use of over-the-counter pain relievers, such as ibuprofen and acetaminophen. These medications can be helpful for mild to moderate pain, but they do not address the underlying cause of neuropathy. In fact, taking too much of these medications can actually damage your nerves.

Another common example is the use of prescription nerve pain medications, such as gabapentin and pregabalin. These medications can be more effective at relieving pain, but they can also cause side effects such as dizziness, drowsiness, and weight gain.

While medications can play a role in managing neuropathy symptoms, it's essential to be realistic about their limitations. Medications cannot cure neuropathy, and they should not be used as a sole solution.

Instead of relying solely on medications, let's look at these steps to broaden our view and explore the various treatment options available for conquering neuropathy:

1. **Acknowledge the complexity**: It's important to grasp that neuropathy is a multi-layered condition. It's unlikely that a single pill will provide a one-size-fits-all solution. A comprehensive approach is key.
2. **Partner with the Right Provider**: Choosing a healthcare provider you trust is crucial for any health journey, especially when dealing with a complex condition. Look for a team who emphasizes individualized care and offers a variety of non-surgical treatment options. At Optimal Performance Chiropractic, we believe in a holistic, collaborative approach to create personalized care plans that address your unique needs and goals.

3. **Integrated treatment:** Consider a blend of approaches. This could include a mix of medication, physical therapy, and lifestyle changes. This multifaceted strategy addresses neuropathy from multiple angles, maximizing your chances of success.

4. **Be open to innovation:** Look for cutting-edge solutions like the RESTORE healing framework for neuropathy. Our innovative approach offers a holistic perspective, combining advanced techniques to tackle neuropathy comprehensively.

Remember, there's no one-size-fits-all solution. By acknowledging the complexity, consulting experienced providers, embracing a combination of treatments, and being open to innovative approaches, you're taking significant strides towards a pain-free, thriving life.

The "Diabetes Only" Myth

The misconception that only people with diabetes develop neuropathy is a widespread one, holding many back from seeking early diagnosis and effective treatment.

While it's true that diabetes is a major risk factor, it's crucial to understand that neuropathy can affect anyone, regardless of their blood sugar levels. Let's debunk this myth and explore the diverse landscape of causes for this condition.

Beyond the Sugar Spike

While uncontrolled diabetes, leading to high blood sugar, can damage nerves, it's far from the only culprit. Here's a glimpse into the diverse world of neuropathy triggers:

- **Autoimmune diseases:** Conditions like lupus, rheumatoid arthritis, and Sjogren's syndrome can attack the nerves, causing neuropathy.
- **Infections:** Viruses, bacteria, and even shingles can damage nerves, leading to temporary or permanent neuropathy.
- **Traumatic injuries:** Accidents, falls, and repetitive stress can injure nerves, triggering neuropathy symptoms.
- **Vitamin deficiencies:** Vitamin B12, B6, and E deficiencies can contribute to nerve damage and neuropathy.
- **Toxins:** Exposure to heavy metals, alcohol, and certain medications can be toxic to nerves, causing neuropathy.
- **Inherited conditions:** Some forms of neuropathy, like Charcot-Marie-Tooth disease, are genetic and affect individuals from birth.

The Importance of Early Recognition:

Ignoring any type of neuropathy, regardless of its cause, can lead to further nerve damage and worsening symptoms. Early diagnosis and intervention are crucial for managing the condition effectively, preserving nerve function, and maintaining quality of life.

Remember:

- Neuropathy isn't just a "diabetic" condition. It's a diverse umbrella term encompassing nerve damage with various causes.
- Unexplained pain, numbness, or tingling in your hands, feet, or elsewhere shouldn't be ignored. Seek a healthcare professional for a proper diagnosis and personalized treatment plan.
- Early intervention matters. Don't let myths cloud your understanding and potentially delay critical action toward managing your health.

By shattering the myth of "diabetes-only" neuropathy, we empower individuals to recognize the broader spectrum of causes, seek timely diagnosis, and embrace effective treatment, leading them on the path to living well with neuropathy.

Beyond Tingles: The Hidden Symptoms of Neuropathy

When it comes to neuropathy, many associate it solely with tingling, numbness, and shooting pains, often in the hands and feet. While these are certainly common symptoms, they represent just a glimpse into the wide and sometimes surprising spectrum of ways neuropathy can manifest. Let's dive deeper and unveil the hidden symptoms that might be whispering clues about underlying nerve damage.

Beyond the Obvious:

While tingling, numbness, and pain are frequently reported, neuropathy can present with a far more diverse set of symptoms, depending on the affected nerves and the severity of the damage. Here are some lesser-known signs to watch out for:

- **Muscle weakness:** Difficulty gripping objects, lifting your foot, or performing everyday tasks like buttoning your shirt could signal weakened muscles due to nerve damage.
- **Balance problems and falls:** Damaged nerves in your legs can affect proprioception (your sense of body position), leading to unsteady gait and increased risk of falls.

- **Digestive issues:** Impaired nerve function in your gut can impact digestion, causing bloating, constipation, or diarrhea.
- **Bladder and bowel dysfunction:** Difficulty controlling your bladder or bowels can occur due to nerve damage affecting these systems.
- **Sexual dysfunction:** Erectile dysfunction in men and decreased libido in both men and women can be related to neuropathy affecting nerves involved in sexual function.
- **Changes in sweating:** Excessive sweating or the inability to sweat in specific areas can be signs of nerve damage impacting sweat glands.
- **Sensitivity to touch or temperature:** Some people with neuropathy experience extreme sensitivity to touch or temperature, even finding light clothing or lukewarm water unbearable.

The Importance of Holistic Awareness:

Recognizing these varied symptoms is crucial because early diagnosis and treatment of neuropathy can help prevent further nerve damage and improve quality of life.

Don't dismiss seemingly unrelated symptoms – they

could be valuable pieces of the puzzle leading to proper diagnosis and effective management.

Remember:

- Neuropathy symptoms extend far beyond tingling and numbness. Watch out for weakness, balance issues, digestive troubles, and other seemingly unrelated signs.
- Consulting a healthcare professional for a comprehensive evaluation is vital if you experience any persistent or concerning symptoms.
- Early diagnosis and intervention can make a significant difference in managing neuropathy and preserving your well-being.

By understanding the diverse and sometimes hidden symptoms of neuropathy, you can empower yourself to advocate for your health and seek timely diagnosis, paving the way for effective treatment and a brighter future. Don't let the "tingling myth" limit your awareness – open your eyes to the broader picture and take charge of your health.

Demystifying the Maze: Navigating Information Overload about Neuropathy

Living with neuropathy can be overwhelming, and the vast amount of information available online can feel like a confusing maze. Sorting through fact and fiction can be challenging, leaving you unsure where to turn for reliable guidance.

So, let's equip you with the tools to navigate this information overload and confidently pursue evidence-based solutions for managing your neuropathy.

Understanding the Landscape

The internet offers a wealth of information, but it's crucial to approach it with a discerning eye. Here are some key points to remember:

- **Not all sources are created equal**: Medical websites, government health agencies, and reputable medical organizations like the Mayo Clinic typically provide trustworthy information. Here are links to a few others:
    - MedlinePlus
    - Department of Health and Human Services (HHS)
    - Centers for Disease Control and Prevention (CDC)

- American Medical Association (AMA)
- National Institutes of Health (NIH)

Be cautious of personal blogs, unverified forums, and sensationalized articles. And please note that while these sources are generally considered reliable, it's always a good idea to discuss any health-related information you find with your doctor. We can help you understand how it applies to your personal situation.

- **Beware of miracle cures and quick fixes**: If something sounds too good to be true, it probably is. Steer clear of claims promising instant relief or one-size-fits-all solutions.
- **Fact-check and verify**: Don't blindly accept information at face value. Cross-reference claims with multiple credible sources and consult healthcare professionals for expert insights.

Developing Your Navigation Skills

Here are some practical tips to help you navigate the information landscape effectively:

- **Ask questions**: Don't hesitate to ask your doctor, therapist, or other healthcare professionals about any information you encounter, especially if it seems confusing or contradictory.

- **Seek reliable communities:** Connect with patient support groups or online forums affiliated with reputable organizations. These communities can offer valuable insights and shared experiences, but remember to approach them with a critical eye as well.
- **Develop critical thinking skills:** Learn to evaluate information objectively. Consider the source, evidence, and potential biases before accepting anything as fact.

Remember:

- **Knowledge is power:** By cultivating critical thinking skills and seeking reliable sources, you empower yourself to make informed decisions about your health and treatment options.
- **Individualized approach:** What works for one person might not work for another. Work with your healthcare team to create a personalized treatment plan based on your unique needs and circumstances.
- **Empowerment through understanding:** By navigating the information landscape

effectively, you gain control over your health journey and can confidently explore different avenues for managing your neuropathy.

You can transform the overwhelming maze into a clear path toward informed decision-making and well-being by approaching information with a discerning eye and seeking guidance from trusted sources. Remember, you are not alone in this journey – equip yourself with knowledge and navigate the information landscape with confidence!

ACTION STEP: Take our free Nerve Damage Evaluation by scanning this code:

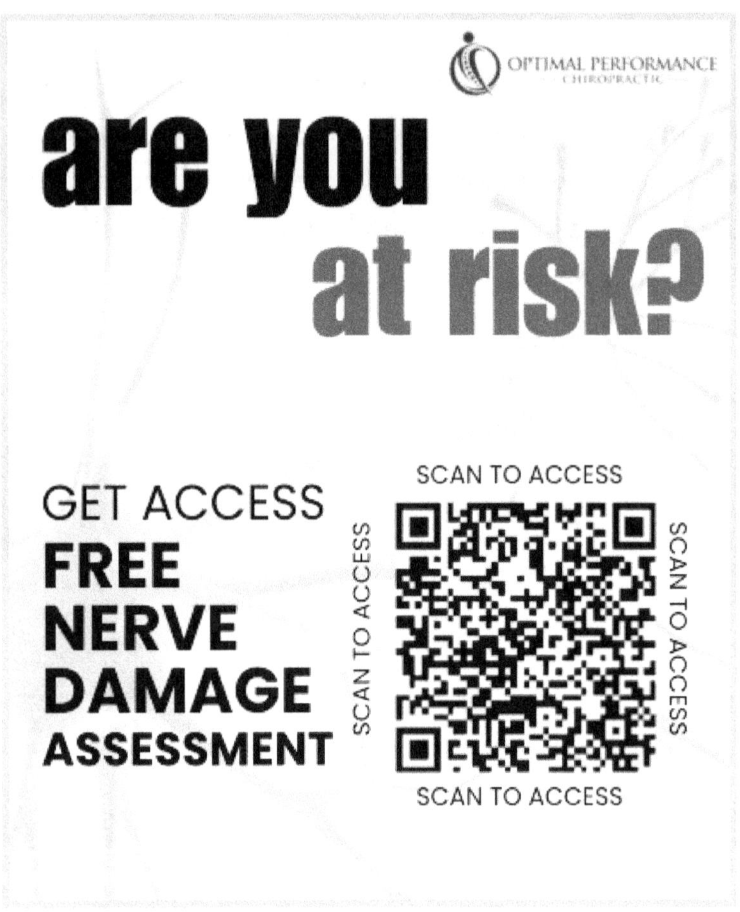

Unlock Your Path to Neuropathy Relief Now: Dial (951) 405-8868 to Speak With Us Today!

8

YOUR NERVOUS SYSTEM: THE BODY'S COMMUNICATION NETWORK

One of my patients, a vibrant woman named Maria, was struggling with a particularly perplexing case of neuropathy. Her symptoms were inconsistent, sometimes flaring up intensely, other times receding into a dull ache. She felt like her body was betraying her, a complex machine gone haywire.

"Dr. Landry," she said, her brow furrowed with worry, "I feel like I'm losing control. My body just isn't doing what it's supposed to anymore."

To help Maria understand, I explained her nervous system as a vast communication network, with nerves acting like intricate wires carrying vital messages throughout her body. Neuropathy, I told her, was like interference on those lines, disrupting the flow of information and leading to the unpredictable symptoms she was experiencing.

This analogy, so simple yet powerful, was a turning point for Maria. It gave her a sense of understanding and control, empowering her to see her body not as an enemy, but as a complex system that could be supported and healed. Of course, every case of neuropathy is unique, and individual results can vary. But understanding the nervous system is a crucial step towards reclaiming your health, just as Maria did.

Imagine your nervous system as a vast information superhighway, buzzing with signals that control every single function in your body. From the way you walk and talk, to the digestion of your food, and even the beating of your heart – your nerves are the messengers making it all happen.

Unfortunately, neuropathy throws a wrench into this finely tuned communication network. Think of it like damaged wires causing short circuits. Those signals that should be traveling smoothly get scrambled, leading to the burning, tingling, or numbness you experience in your feet, legs, or hands. But neuropathy's impact doesn't stop there.

This disruption can impact your balance, making walking difficult. It can interfere with your digestion, causing uncomfortable bloating or other issues. Even your sleep can suffer as those nerve signals keep misfiring, making it tough to get the rest you need.

The good news? Your body possesses an incredible capacity to heal itself. That's true for your nervous system as well. While neuropathy can feel overwhelmingly complex, the RESTORE approach focuses on harnessing your body's innate healing potential, fostering an environment where damaged nerves can begin to regenerate and function can be restored.

Decoding the Nervous System

Let's break down your nervous system so you can better understand how neuropathy affects it. It's helpful to think of it in two main parts:

1. **The Central Nervous System (CNS):** This is your body's command center – the brain and spinal cord. They process information, generate thoughts and emotions, and send out instructions to the rest of your body.

2. **The Peripheral Nervous System (PNS):** Imagine your PNS as a massive network of wires branching out from

your spinal cord, connecting your CNS to every organ, muscle, and tissue. It's responsible for things like sensation (touch, temperature), movement, and even some automatic functions like your heart rate. Neuropathy primarily targets this peripheral system.

Now, let's zoom in on an individual nerve. It's like a tiny insulated cable. The core wire that carries the message is called the axon. Surrounding that axon is a protective layer called the myelin sheath – think of it like the rubber insulation around an electrical wire.

When neuropathy strikes, it can damage both the axon and the myelin sheath. With damaged insulation, signals get garbled, leading to pain. Or the "wire" itself is broken, causing numbness. These damaged nerves are why you experience those frustrating neuropathy symptoms.

When Things Go Wrong: How Neuropathy Develops

Unfortunately, things can go wrong with those incredible communication networks we call nerves. This brings us to neuropathy, which comes in a few different flavors:

- **Peripheral Neuropathy:** This is our main focus. It's when the nerves in those outer limbs – your feet, hands, legs, and sometimes arms – become damaged. This is what leads to all those uncomfortable tingling, burning, and numb sensations.
- **Autonomic Neuropathy:** This type affects the nerves controlling automatic functions within our body – things like digestion, heart rate, and blood pressure. While less common, it's important to be aware of.

So, why does neuropathy happen? It's rarely a single culprit. Instead, it's usually a combination of factors that create a domino effect of damage. Let's look at some of the biggest pieces of that puzzle:

- **Unstable Blood Sugar:** Blood sugar spikes and crashes throw your entire body out of whack, including your nerves.
- **Inflammation:** Think of this as a fire raging throughout your body. Nerves are especially vulnerable to this inflammatory damage.
- **Nutritional Deficiencies:** Nerves need specific vitamins and minerals to function correctly and repair themselves. When your diet falls short, so does your nerve health.

- **Other Medical Conditions:** Diabetes is the most well-known risk factor, but neuropathy goes hand-in-hand with issues like autoimmune disorders, thyroid problems, and even past infections or toxins.

The key takeaway? To truly conquer neuropathy, we need to go beyond just covering up symptoms. We need to dig deep to identify and address those root causes.

Harnessing the Body's Healing Power

Here's the incredibly good news: Your body isn't a static machine. It has a remarkable ability to heal, and that includes your nerves. This is where a concept called neuroplasticity comes in.

Neuroplasticity means your brain and nerves can change, adapt, and form new connections. Think of it like rewiring a damaged circuit board. While this doesn't happen overnight, it's the foundation of true healing for neuropathy.

So, how do we support this natural healing process? Let's break it down:

- **Specific Nutrients:** Your nerves are hungry for B vitamins, magnesium, and other key nutrients. These act as building blocks for repair and protect against further damage.

- **Lifestyle Adjustments:** Simple things like getting restorative sleep, managing stress, and the right types of movement all reduce inflammation and create a better environment for your nerves to heal.
- **The RESTORE Approach:** Our therapies are designed to directly stimulate nerve regeneration, increase blood flow to damaged areas, and calm that "fire" of inflammation. Combined with targeted nutrition and those lifestyle shifts, this creates a powerful synergy for healing.

It's important to remember that healing takes time and consistency. But by understanding and actively supporting your body's innate healing mechanisms, you unlock the potential for real, lasting improvement in your neuropathy.

Beyond the Physical: The Mind-Body Connection

We often think of healing in purely physical terms, but when it comes to neuropathy, we can't ignore the mind-body connection. Let's dive into why this matters.

Stress – The Hidden Enemy

When you're constantly stressed, your body is in a chronic "fight or flight" mode. This floods your system with stress hormones, worsens inflammation, and ultimately makes your neuropathy symptoms flare up. Plus, it keeps you in a state where healing simply can't be a priority.

Stress Relief: Key to Healing

Finding ways to manage stress isn't just about feeling better in the moment, it's about unlocking your body's ability to heal. Here are some techniques well-suited for those with neuropathy:

- **Mindfulness Practices**: Simple focusing exercises, like noticing your breath for a few minutes, can pull you into the present and calm a racing mind.
- **Gentle Movement**: Yoga, Tai Chi, or simply mindful walking can be great ways to release tension and improve circulation.
- **Guided Relaxation**: There are many apps or audio recordings offering guided meditations, helping you shift into a more relaxed state.

The key is finding what works for you. Even 5-10

minutes of these practices daily can make a significant difference over time.

The Power of Positive Mindset

You might think positive mindset is just feel-good fluff, but when it comes to neuropathy, it's much more powerful than that.

The Self-Fulfilling Prophecy

If you believe your neuropathy has you trapped, and that it will only get worse, those thoughts become a roadblock to progress. However, when you cultivate the belief that healing IS possible, you're more likely to embrace the RESTORE program wholeheartedly.

Mind Over Matter

A Positive mindset won't magically erase your neuropathy overnight. However, it reduces stress (which we know hinders healing), increases motivation, and empowers you to face challenges with greater resilience.

Hope Is Fuel

The healing journey can be long. Belief in your body's ability to improve and faith in the RESTORE process can make all the difference in staying committed, even when progress feels slow.

It's important to be honest about the challenges, but don't let fear or past disappointments steal your hope. Empower yourself by focusing on the potential for a better tomorrow.

By now, you have a much deeper understanding of how your amazing nervous system works and the ways that neuropathy disrupts its delicate balance. This knowledge isn't just about knowing the facts; it's about empowerment. The more you understand, the clearer it becomes that you're not just a victim of this condition; you're an active participant in your healing journey.

RESTORE is designed to be a partnership. It honors the complexity of neuropathy by addressing not just the physical damage, but the mental, emotional, and lifestyle factors that so greatly impact your overall nervous system health.

Think of it this way: If your nerves are that intricate communication network, we're providing the tools to repair the wires, boost the signal quality, and even teach your brain and body healthier communication patterns. This multi-pronged approach is what sets RESTORE apart, offering true holistic healing and the best chance of lasting relief from neuropathy.

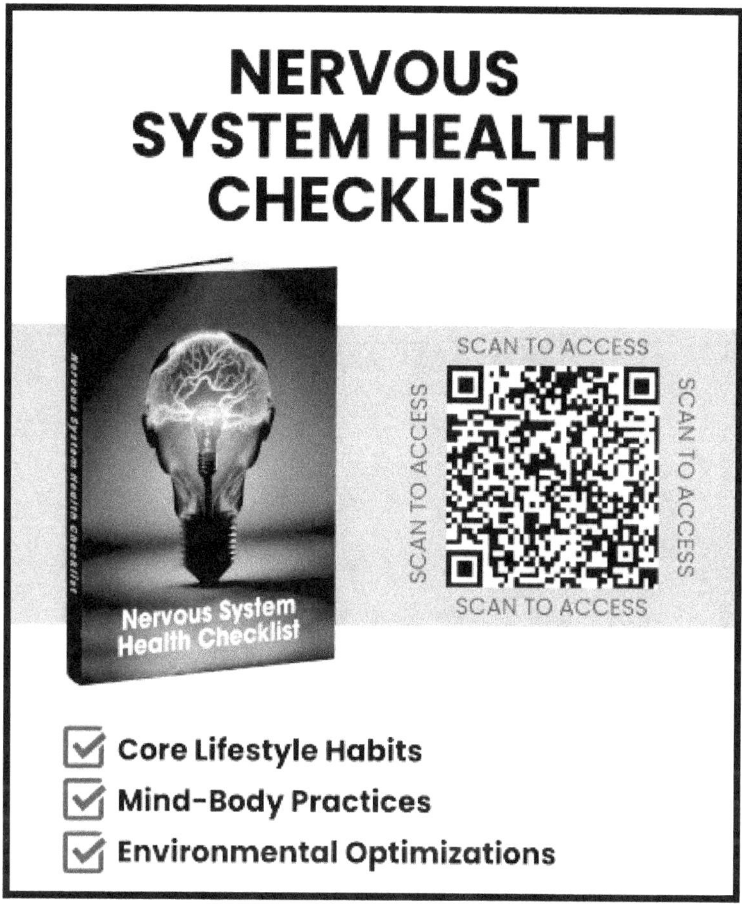

Unlock Your Path to Neuropathy Relief Now: Dial (951) 405-8868 to Speak With Us Today!

9

———

STATINS & NEUROPATHY: A CLOSER LOOK AT THE RISKS

If you, like millions of Americans, have been told you need a statin medication to lower your cholesterol, it's important to understand what that decision truly means. Statins are among the most widely prescribed drugs in the world, making them a critical topic for anyone battling chronic health issues like neuropathy.

For years, the message on cholesterol has been simple: high cholesterol is bad, and lowering it at nearly any cost is good. However, a growing body of research paints a much more complicated picture. It forces us to ask: Are the benefits of statins always worth the potential risks?

This question is especially urgent for those struggling with neuropathy. Studies show a clear link between statin use and an increased risk of developing neuropathy, or worsening of existing symptoms. Unfortunately, many patients (and even some doctors) are unaware of this potential side effect. This chapter aims to give you the knowledge to make informed choices about your health.

How Statins Work (And How They Can Harm)

Let's break down how statins actually work inside your body, and why, despite their intended purpose, they can end up doing more harm than good.

How Statins Lower Cholesterol: Your liver is your body's cholesterol factory. Statins work by essentially slowing down this factory's production line. Seems like a good thing if your numbers are high, right? Well, it's not quite that simple.

The CoQ10 Problem: Your liver doesn't just make cholesterol. It also creates something called CoQ10, which is absolutely crucial for energy production in every single cell. Think of CoQ10 as the fuel for your cellular power plants. Here's the catch: Statins block the same pathway that makes CoQ10, meaning lower cholesterol often comes at the price of depleted CoQ10.

Why CoQ10 Matters for Your Nerves: Your nerves and muscles are incredibly energy-hungry. Depleting their fuel source (CoQ10) can lead to the very kinds of symptoms seen in neuropathy – weakness, pain, fatigue, and more.

Side Effects Beyond Neuropathy: We can't talk about statins without mentioning the broader range of problems reported by those taking them. This includes muscle aches, cognitive fog, blood sugar disruptions, and even increased risk for conditions like Parkinson's and liver damage. While some dismiss these as "mild," they have a massive impact on quality of life – especially when you're already facing a condition like neuropathy.

Statins & Neuropathy: What the Research Says

Unfortunately, research makes it clear – statins and neuropathy are more connected than many patients realize. Let's look at the evidence, and why this demands extra caution in making treatment decisions.

Who's Most at Risk?

Certain factors make statin-induced neuropathy more likely:

- **Existing Neuropathy or Diabetes:** If your nerves are already vulnerable, statins can make them even more susceptible to damage.

- **Older Age:** Our bodies become less efficient at processing medication over time, increasing the chance of side effects.
- **Taking Multiple Medications:** Certain drugs interact with statins, raising the risk of complications.
- **Vitamin D Deficiency:** Low Vitamin D levels may compound the nerve-damaging effects of statins.

The Misdiagnosis Problem

Imagine this scenario: You're taking a statin, and gradually your neuropathy symptoms worsen – more burning in your feet, increased weakness, and it's harder to walk. Most people (and even many doctors) assume this means the disease is simply progressing. This can lead to:

- **Upping the Statin Dose:** The logic is, "If cholesterol is the problem, and it's not coming down enough, we need more medication." Unfortunately, this often intensifies the side effects.
- **Adding Other Medications:** Doctors might prescribe additional drugs focused on nerve pain, not realizing the statin itself could be fueling the fire.

- **Unnecessary Anxiety:** Thinking their condition is spiraling out of control adds mental and emotional burdens on top of the physical ones.

Here's where it gets even trickier: Some patients with statin-induced neuropathy actually DO experience a period of initial improvement on the medication, as their cholesterol numbers fall. This can lull them into a false sense of security, masking the damage the statin is doing longer-term.

The key takeaway? If you're on a statin and ANY change in your neuropathy symptoms occurs – better or worse – it warrants a deeper conversation with your doctor. Don't assume every setback is inevitable disease progression.

Why Open Discussions Matter

The decision to take statins or not is complex. Your doctor needs to weigh your individual heart health risks with the potential for serious side effects like neuropathy. It's a conversation about quality vs. quantity of life, and YOUR input should be central.

Natural Alternatives for Heart Health

Here's the good news: protecting your heart health doesn't have to mean relying solely on medications like statins. Natural approaches provide a powerful, multifaceted way to support your cardiovascular system AND reduce the very things that drive neuropathy progression.

Beyond Cholesterol

Think of inflammation like a fire raging inside your blood vessels. Over time, this causes damage to the delicate lining, making them rough and sticky. This is where cholesterol has its chance to build up, potentially forming those dangerous plaques that can lead to heart attack or stroke. Statins put a temporary band-aid on high cholesterol numbers, but don't extinguish the underlying fire.

Oxidative damage is another key player. Imagine all your cells, including those lining your blood vessels, as constantly producing 'exhaust fumes' from their energy production processes. Antioxidants are like your body's air filtration system, neutralizing those fumes. Excess inflammation and an unhealthy lifestyle can overload the system, essentially 'rusting' your blood vessels from the inside out.

Why does this matter for neuropathy? Your nerves are particularly sensitive to both inflammation and oxidative damage. The same things that put your heart at risk are contributing to the breakdown of your nerves as well. Addressing these root issues isn't just about protecting your heart – it's about safeguarding your entire body, and especially those vulnerable nerves.

Lifestyle as Your Best Medicine

Let's emphasize how powerful lifestyle shifts can be in protecting your heart and nerves. Start with prioritizing an anti-inflammatory diet. This means ditching processed junk and filling your plate with vibrant, whole foods. Think of all those colorful fruits and vegetables as an army of antioxidants, safeguarding your blood vessels and nerves. It's also crucial to choose foods that won't send your blood sugar soaring, as those spikes cause widespread damage – especially to sensitive nerves.

Don't underestimate the power of movement – even if your neuropathy creates limitations. Find what works for you, whether it's short walks, chair-based exercise, or gentle water exercises like water aerobics. Moving your body boosts circulation (so important for those healing nerves) and helps your body combat chronic inflammation.

Lastly, remember that stress relief isn't a luxury, it's a necessity. When you're constantly in "fight or flight" mode, stress hormones surge, harming both your heart and nerves. Simple mindfulness practices, deep breathing, or even taking a few minutes for a relaxing hobby, can make a substantial difference when done consistently.

Supplements: A Targeted Approach

While a healthy diet and lifestyle are foundational, targeted supplements can supercharge your heart and nerve protection. First up are omega-3 fatty acids, found in fish oil. These are superstars when it comes to taming inflammation, benefiting both your blood vessels and those sensitive nerves.

Certain nutrients act like your body's internal blood sugar management team. Magnesium and alpha-lipoic acid are key players, helping to keep blood sugar levels steady and preventing those harmful spikes that contribute to neuropathy.

Lastly, antioxidants are your shield against that internal "rust" we call oxidative damage. Resveratrol (found in grapes and red wine), turmeric (that bright yellow spice), and many others each provide unique protective benefits for your heart and circulatory system.

Important Note: Supplements are most effective when combined with those healthy lifestyle changes. Before adding any, always talk to your doctor, especially if you take other medications.

Making Informed Decisions

This chapter isn't about scaring you away from statins, but about making sure you have all the information to make the best possible decisions for YOUR health. Let's discuss how to navigate this, whether you're currently on statins or considering starting them.

Don't Go It Alone: If you take statins, stopping abruptly can be dangerous. Cholesterol rebound is a real risk, and it's essential to do so under your doctor's supervision. This may involve a gradual taper or exploring alternatives.

Questions to Spark Conversation

Your next appointment shouldn't be a passive checkup. Here are a few questions to advocate for yourself:

- "What are my specific heart risks, and how does this statin help lower them?"
- "Are there lifestyle changes I could make to potentially reduce my need for medication?"
- "If I experience any new muscle pain,

weakness, or cognitive changes, should I report them immediately?"

- "Can we discuss non-statin options for cholesterol, and their pros and cons?"

Sometimes, statins may be necessary. But even then, the RESTORE approach is vital. By addressing inflammation, blood sugar, etc., you're protecting your heart and nerves, and minimizing the potential damage statins can cause over time. It's about smart, integrative care, not one-size-fits-all prescriptions.

This chapter isn't about scaring you away from statins, but about making sure you have all the information to make the best possible decisions for YOUR health. It's a conversation about quality vs. quantity of life, and YOUR input should be central.

Consider the experience of John, who reached out to me after months of increasing neuropathy symptoms. "I was put on a statin for my heart," he explained, "and my doctor said the tingling and numbness in my feet were just part of my neuropathy progressing. But it was getting so bad I could barely walk."

John's story, while individual results may vary, highlights a crucial point: don't assume every change in your neuropathy is inevitable disease progression. Statins can be a contributing factor, and open communication with your doctor about both the risks and benefits is essential. Remember, true health encompasses thriving nerves, a strong heart, AND a life where you feel your best.

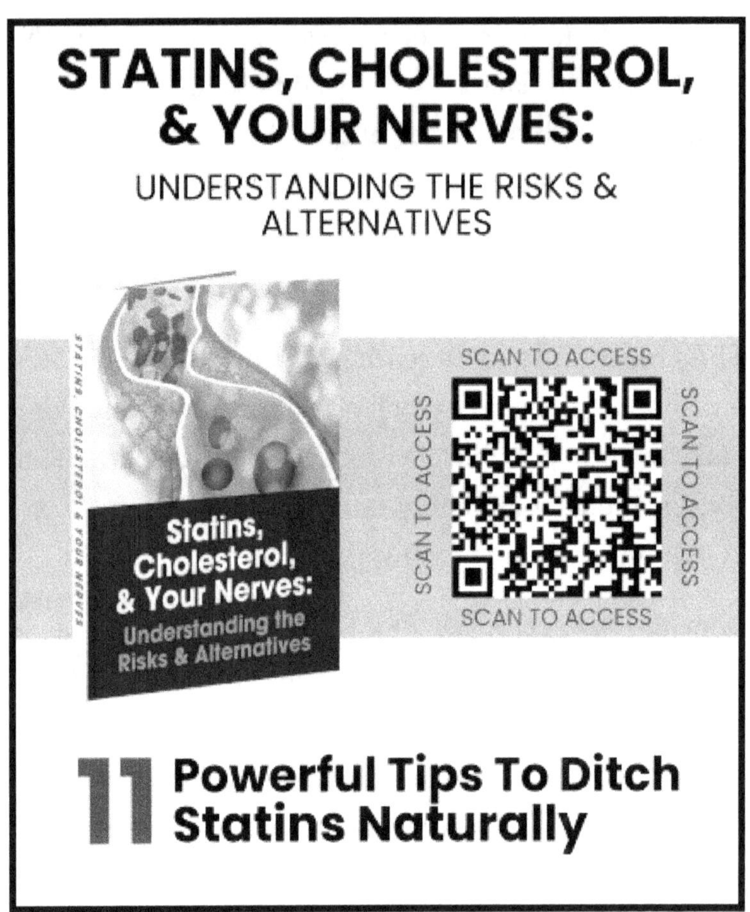

Unlock Your Path to Neuropathy Relief Now: Dial (951) 405-8868 to Speak With Us Today!

10

———

THE RESTORE BLUEPRINT: UNLOCKING NEUROPATHY HEALING

Neuropathy can rob us of the simple joys of life, making every step a challenge and every touch a torment. Our RESTORE healing framework for neuropathy is built on the belief that the body has an innate ability to heal itself. At Optimal Performance Chiropractic, we have carefully crafted a holistic approach that nourishes this natural healing power, allowing it to flourish and guide you on a path to wellness.

With deep respect for the human body and its intricate workings, our neuropathy program not only offers healing from neuropathy but also the possibility of THRIVING. In this chapter, we'll explore the RESTORE healing framework for neuropathy and what each letter represents.

R - Remove Toxins

Toxins lurk in surprising places. They're in the air we breathe, the food we eat, and even the products we use. Some of the most common culprits that can harm nerves include:

- **Heavy Metals:** Things like lead, mercury, and arsenic can accumulate in our bodies over time. Sources can include old paint, contaminated water, and certain fish.
- **Pesticides & Herbicides:** Exposure to these chemicals through food or the environment can cause nerve damage.
- **Industrial Chemicals:** Found in cleaning products, plastics, and even personal care items, these substances can disrupt nerve function.
- **Metabolic Byproducts:** Our bodies naturally produce waste products, but an unhealthy lifestyle and poor diet can lead to excessive buildup, potentially impacting nerves.

The Detox Strategy

Removing toxins is an essential first step in the healing process. Here's how we'll approach it:

1. **Identifying Sources:** We'll review your lifestyle, diet, and environment to pinpoint potential sources of toxin exposure. This might involve some detective work!

2. **Reducing Exposure:** We'll create a plan to minimize your contact with harmful substances. This could include switching to organic food, using natural cleaning products, and filtering your water.

3. **Supporting Detoxification Organs:** Your liver, kidneys, and lymphatic system are your body's natural toxin filters. We'll focus on dietary and lifestyle changes that bolster their function, helping your body flush out harmful substances.

Important Note: Detoxification should be approached thoughtfully. Sudden, drastic detoxes can be overwhelming for your body. We will create a safe and customized plan tailored to your needs.

E- Enhance Nutrition

Your nerves depend on a steady supply of crucial nutrients to thrive. Sadly, the standard modern diet often falls short of these essential elements. We'll work to correct this through strategic food choices. Here's what we'll focus on:

- **Antioxidants:** These powerful compounds fight inflammation and protect nerves from oxidative damage. Think of them as your nerves' personal defense system. We'll focus on vibrantly colored fruits and vegetables like berries, leafy greens, and bell peppers.

- **B vitamins:** The B-complex vitamins, particularly B1, B6, and B12, are vital for nerve health. They help build and repair the protective myelin sheath around your nerves and support healthy nerve signaling. Excellent sources include leafy greens, eggs, and lean meats.

- **Omega-3 Fatty Acids:** These healthy fats have anti-inflammatory properties and support nerve cell communication. We'll focus on sources like fatty fish (salmon, tuna), walnuts, and flaxseeds.

- **Magnesium:** This essential mineral helps relax nerves and reduce pain signals. Leafy greens, nuts, seeds, and whole grains are excellent sources.

- **Alpha-Lipoic Acid (ALA):** This potent antioxidant helps protect nerves and may even promote regeneration. You'll find it in spinach, broccoli, and organ meats.

Beyond Just Food

Sometimes, even with a healthy diet, you might need a boost. In these cases, I may recommend targeted supplements to address any specific deficiencies and accelerate the healing process.

It's About More Than Single Nutrients

While these key nutrients are vital, we'll look at your overall dietary pattern. An anti-inflammatory, whole-foods diet is the foundation for healthy nerves. We'll create a plan that's enjoyable, sustainable, and packed with healing goodness.

S - Stimulate Circulation

Think of your blood vessels like highways delivering essential supplies to your nerves. When circulation is poor, it's like a traffic jam – nutrients and oxygen can't efficiently reach their destination. This can starve your nerves, leading to further damage and contributing to the pain and discomfort of neuropathy.

Here's how we'll address circulation:

1. **Exercise:** Regular, gentle exercise is one of the best ways to improve blood flow throughout your body. We'll design an exercise program that's appropriate for your fitness level and

enjoyable, focusing on activities like walking, swimming, and gentle yoga.

2. **Targeted Therapies:** In addition to general exercise, specific therapies can help increase circulation to your extremities. These might include massage techniques, compression therapy, or even specialized treatments like vibration therapy.

3. **Elevation:** A simple but effective strategy is to elevate your legs when resting. This helps reduce any swelling and promotes better blood flow back towards your heart.

4. **Hydration:** Staying properly hydrated is crucial for maintaining healthy blood volume and circulation. We'll discuss ways to ensure you're getting enough water throughout the day.

5. **Addressing Underlying Issues:** Sometimes, poor circulation is a symptom of other health conditions like diabetes or vascular disease. If necessary, I'll collaborate with other healthcare providers to manage any underlying factors impacting your blood flow.

The Benefits of Enhanced Circulation

By improving circulation, we can:

- **Deliver Oxygen & Nutrients:** Provide your nerves with the resources they desperately need for repair and regeneration.
- **Reduce Inflammation:** Healthy blood flow helps remove inflammatory waste products that contribute to nerve pain.
- **Promote Healing:** Better circulation sets the stage for your nerves to heal and function optimally.
- **Ease Symptoms:** Improved circulation can contribute to decreased pain, numbness, and tingling associated with neuropathy.

T - Transform Habits

Many seemingly ordinary habits can put a strain on your nerves, exacerbating neuropathy symptoms. Here are some common culprits:

- **Poor Posture:** Slouching or hunching for prolonged periods compresses nerves, particularly in the neck and shoulders. This can lead to pain, numbness, and tingling.

- **Sedentary Lifestyle:** Inactivity weakens your muscles and reduces blood flow, making nerves more vulnerable to damage.
- **High Blood Sugar:** Uncontrolled blood sugar levels, which can be related to diet and lifestyle, directly damage nerves over time.
- **Smoking:** The toxins in cigarette smoke harm blood vessels and restrict oxygen flow to nerves.
- **Excessive Alcohol Consumption:** Alcohol can be neurotoxic, directly damaging nerves.
- **Stress:** Chronic stress releases inflammatory chemicals and disrupts nerve function.
- **Sleep Deprivation:** Not getting sufficient restorative sleep hinders your body's natural healing processes, including nerve repair.

The Transformative Process

Here's how we'll approach habit transformation for healthier nerves:

1. **Assessment:** We'll start with a thorough evaluation of your daily routines. Together, we'll pinpoint habits that might be hindering your progress.
2. **Awareness is Key:** The first step towards change is recognizing areas where adjustments

can have a big impact. I'll help you develop a heightened awareness of how your habits influence your nerves.

3. **Small, Sustainable Changes**: We'll focus on making gradual, achievable shifts in your daily life. This might include simple posture changes, incorporating short activity breaks, trying stress-management techniques, or improving your sleep environment.

4. **Support and Accountability**: I'll be your guide, offering tips, resources, and encouragement throughout your habit transformation journey.

The Benefits of Healthier Habits

By changing harmful habits, you can:

- **Reduce Nerve Stress**: Minimize direct strain and pressure on your nerves.
- **Improve Overall Health**: Many healthy habits benefit not just your nerves but your overall well-being.
- **Enhance Healing**: Creating a supportive environment allows your body to focus on nerve regeneration.
- **Empowerment**: Taking control of your habits

is empowering and promotes a sense of control over your health.

O - Optimize Nerve Function

Your nerves are like electrical wires carrying messages to and from your brain. They transmit signals about pain, temperature, and touch, and control body processes like muscle movement. Neuropathy can disrupt this communication, leading to pain, numbness, tingling, and weakness.

Here are some approaches we might use, tailored to your specific needs:

- **Manual Therapies:** Techniques like specialized massage, stretching, and gentle joint manipulation can improve nerve mobility, reduce stiffness, and increase blood flow to the affected areas.
- **Neurological Re-education:** Specific exercises and protocols can help 'rewire' the communication between your brain and affected nerves, potentially improving sensation and reducing pain signals.
- **Electrical Stimulation:** Therapies like TENS (Transcutaneous Electrical Nerve Stimulation)

use gentle electrical currents to block pain
signals and promote nerve healing.

- **Light Therapy:** Certain wavelengths of light
(like low-level laser therapy) can stimulate
nerve regeneration and reduce inflammation.
- **Supportive Supplements:** In addition to
dietary changes, specific supplements may
support nerve function and reduce pain.
Examples include alpha-lipoic acid, B-complex
vitamins, and acetyl-l-carnitine.

Important Considerations

- **Individualized Approach:** The best
combination of therapies will depend on your
specific type of neuropathy, the severity of your
symptoms, and your overall health.
- **Nerve Regeneration Takes Time:** These
techniques work to stimulate your body's own
healing potential. While some people
experience rapid relief, know that consistent
effort over time is often key to significant
improvement.

The Goal: Improved Quality of Life

By optimizing nerve function, we strive to:

- **Decrease Pain & Discomfort:** Reduce the intensity and frequency of pain, numbness, and tingling.
- **Improve Sensation:** Help restore feeling and sensitivity in affected areas.
- **Enhance Muscle Strength:** Improve strength and coordination, making daily activities easier.
- **Promote Overall Well-being:** Optimizing nerve health contributes to a better overall quality of life.

R - Revitalize Movement

Moving your body in smart ways offers a host of benefits for those with neuropathy:

- **Boosted Circulation:** As we've discussed, exercise increases blood flow which nourishes your nerves with oxygen and nutrients.
- **Reduced Inflammation:** Regular movement helps decrease inflammation throughout your body, which can directly benefit your nerves.

- **Nerve Regeneration:** Certain types of exercise may stimulate the growth and repair of damaged nerves.
- **Pain Management:** Exercise helps release endorphins, your body's natural painkillers, and can improve your pain tolerance.
- **Improved Balance and Coordination:** Strengthening your muscles and practicing safe movement patterns can reduce the risk of falls and injuries, a common concern with neuropathy.
- **Mental Well-being:** Exercise is a fantastic mood booster and stress reliever, both of which are deeply connected with how we experience pain.

Developing a Safe and Effective Plan

Here's how we'll approach exercise together:

1. **Starting Point Assessment:** We'll evaluate your current fitness level, any pain limitations, and your personal preferences.
2. **Gradual Progression:** We'll start with gentle movements and gradually increase intensity and duration as you become stronger and less bothered by symptoms.

3. **Focus on Form:** Proper form is crucial to prevent further injury and maximize the benefits of exercise. We'll provide detailed instructions and ensure you're moving in a way that's supportive of your nerves.

4. **Variety:** We'll incorporate a mix of exercises, including aerobic activities (like walking or swimming), flexibility exercises, and strength training to target different areas of your body.

5. **Enjoyment Factor:** Finding the movement you enjoy is key to sticking with it! We'll explore different options and find activities that feel good.

It's essential to listen to your body and progress at a pace that feels comfortable. Some discomfort may be expected, but we'll distinguish it from sharp nerve pain and tailor your plan accordingly.

E - Encourage Regeneration

While nerve damage can be frustrating, it's important to know that your nerves have a remarkable ability to heal and regrow. There are two main types of nerves:

- **Peripheral Nerves:** These nerves extend from your spinal cord out into your arms, legs, and the rest of your body. They have a greater capacity to regenerate compared to nerves in the brain and spinal cord.

- **Central Nerves**: These nerves make up your brain and spinal cord. Their regeneration ability is more limited.

Here's how we'll support your nerves' natural healing process:

- **Nutrition as the Foundation**: The "Enhance Nutrition" aspect of the RESTORE framework is vital. Your nerves need the right building blocks (like vitamins, minerals, and antioxidants) to regenerate.
- **Targeted Therapies**: We may incorporate therapies that directly stimulate nerve repair, such as light therapy, electrical stimulation, or specific manual techniques.
- **Reducing Nerve Stress**: Minimizing inflammation, managing blood sugar levels, and addressing any physical compression on your nerves creates an optimal environment for regeneration.
- **Movement is Key**: Gentle, appropriate exercise promotes blood flow and may even release factors that stimulate nerve growth.

- **Mind-Body Connection:** Stress can negatively impact healing. We'll discuss stress-management techniques like mindfulness and guided relaxation to support a calmer nervous system.
- **Supportive Supplementation:** Specific nutrients, like acetyl-l-carnitine and alpha-lipoic acid, might play a role in accelerating nerve regeneration.

Patience and Persistence

Nerve regeneration takes time. While some people might see improvements quickly, for others, it's a slower process. Consistent effort is essential, and celebrating even small victories will keep you motivated!

Unlock Inspiration: View Our Real-Life Victories and Success Stories by scanning the code below:

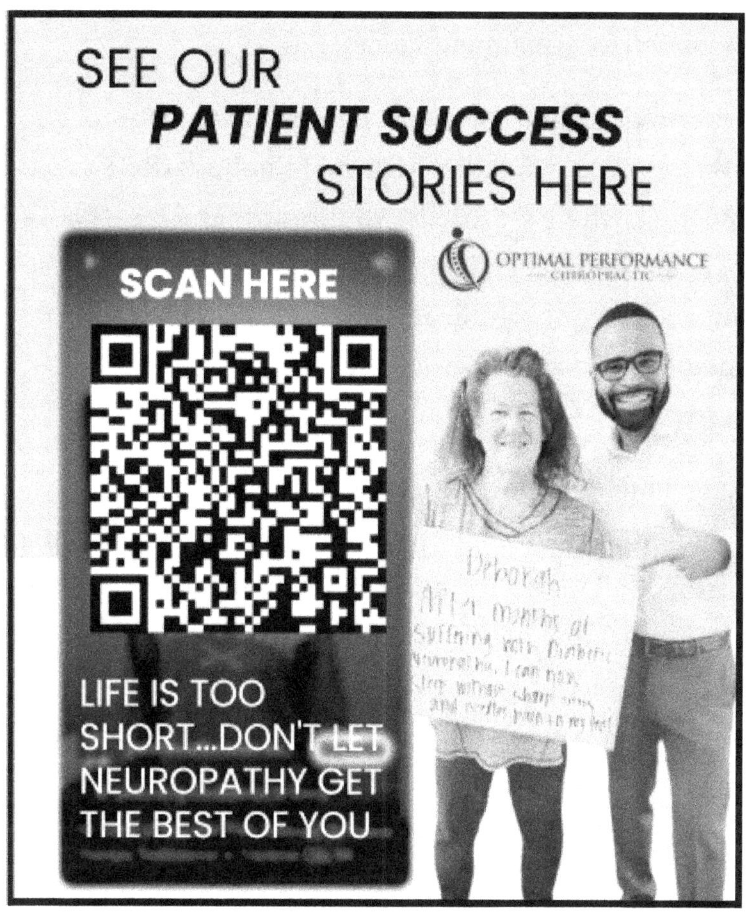

Discover if the RESTORE Neuropathy Program is Right for You

The RESTORE Neuropathy Program offers a comprehensive approach, tailored to your unique needs and goals.

Personalized Treatment Plans

Our program goes beyond a one-size-fits-all approach. We start with a detailed Report of Findings (ROF) meeting, where we discuss your results and create a personalized plan aligned with your health objectives. Your partner or significant other is welcome to join, as their support plays a crucial role in your journey.

Prior to your initial consultation, our dedicated team, which includes doctors, case managers, and rehabilitation specialists, carefully reviews your health history and intake forms. This allows us to understand your individual needs and preferences and to determine if our holistic, non-surgical approach is a good fit for your situation. We prioritize personalized care and strive to create a plan that aligns with your health goals.

Advanced Therapies at Your Fingertips

While not every therapy applies to everyone, we offer a diverse range of options, potentially including:

At-Home Therapies

- **Nerve Stimulation & Rebuilding:** Revitalizes nerves with a state-of-the-art device, reducing pain and numbness.

- **Light Therapy (LLLT):** Stimulates blood flow and healing with powerful infrared and red light.
- **Foot Vibration Therapy:** Improves circulation and balance with gentle foot and calf vibrations.

Nutritional Approach

- **Dietary Changes:** Tailored advice to reduce inflammation and nourish your body.
- **Nutritional Supplementation:** Carefully chosen supplements to combat inflammation, balance pH, and improve blood flow.

In-Clinic Treatments

- **SoftWave TRT:** Promotes healing and pain relief at the cellular level using sound waves.
- **Chiropractic BioPhysics:** Gentle adjustments to relieve nerve pressure and promote regeneration.
- **Foot Levelers Custom Orthotics:** Support all 3 arches of your feet after a custom 3D scan is completed, helping to eliminate foot pain.
- **Balance Tracking Systems:** A non-invasive,

easy-to-use system that measures your balance and fall risk.

What Sets Us Apart

- **Personalized Care:** Tailored treatment plans and a supportive team dedicated to your success.
- **Advanced Technology:** Cutting-edge therapies to maximize your healing potential.
- **Passionate Providers:** We care deeply about your journey and strive for your well-being.

Is RESTORE Right for You?

This program may be ideal if you:

- Are diagnosed with peripheral neuropathy.
- Are seeking non-invasive and drug-free treatment options.
- Desire a personalized approach tailored to your specific needs.
- Are committed to actively participating in your healing journey.
- Are looking for a supportive and encouraging environment.

Ready to Explore Your Options?

Contact us today at (951) 405-8868 or visit our website at optimalperformancechiropractic.com/special to take advantage of our new patient special offer which includes a consultation, exam, x-rays (if necessary), and first treatment. Learn more about how the RESTORE neuropathy program can help you reclaim your life and experience lasting relief by contacting us today. Remember, you're not alone in this journey. Let us guide you towards a brighter future, one step at a time.

Disclaimer: The consultation is for informational purposes and does not guarantee specific results. Treatment plans are personalized based on individual needs, and outcomes may vary. Please consult with our team to determine if our approach is right for you.

Embarking on Your RESTORE Journey: A Beginner's Guide

Let's now discuss the initial steps after joining the RESTORE program and what that would look like so we can set a successful and enriching journey for you.

Laying the Groundwork

- **Gather Your Medical Records:** Compile a comprehensive record of your medical history, diagnoses, medications, and past treatments. This information aids your team in tailoring the program to your unique needs.

- **Schedule Your Evaluation & Report of Findings (ROF):** This crucial meeting involves a detailed review of your medical records and a discussion of your health goals. We will perform various tests to help determine the nature and severity of your nerve damage. If your case is accepted, our team will create a personalized treatment plan aligned with your aspirations. Encourage your partner, spouse, or significant other to attend this meeting, as their support is vital to your success.

- **Review Your Financial Coverage:** Familiarize yourself with your insurance coverage and any potential out-of-pocket expenses associated with the program. Discuss any financial concerns with our team to ensure clarity and transparency.

- **Prepare for Commitment:** The RESTORE program requires active participation and commitment to prescribed therapies, exercises, and lifestyle adjustments. Embracing these efforts is essential to maximize your healing potential. We like to say that this is a 50/50 process. You need to do your part, and we will do ours!

Getting Started

- **Connect with Your Care Team:** Don't hesitate to reach out to your assigned doctor, case manager, or other team members with questions or concerns. We are here to support you every step of the way.
- **Gather Necessary Supplies:** Depending on your personalized treatment plan, you may need to acquire specific equipment like at-home therapy devices or nutritional supplements. We will provide clear instructions and guidance.
- **Explore Resources:** We offer a wealth of educational resources on our website and app, covering various aspects of neuropathy, treatment options, and healthy living tips. Delve into these resources to empower yourself with knowledge.

Remember:

- **Communication is Key:** Open and honest communication with your care team is crucial for monitoring your progress, addressing challenges, and adjusting your program as needed.

- **Celebrate Small Victories**: Acknowledge and celebrate every improvement, no matter how small. These milestones fuel your motivation and reinforce your commitment to your well-being.
- **Be Patient and Persistent**: Healing takes time and dedication. Embrace the journey, trust the process, and stay committed to your personalized program for lasting results.

This program isn't merely about managing symptoms; it seeks to restore, regenerate, and rejuvenate. It's a promise of not just living WITH neuropathy but THRIVING BEYOND IT. That's the fundamental difference and the potential game-changer that sets RESTORE apart from conventional neuropathy treatments.

Just ask Jenny, who after years of struggling with painful neuropathy, decided to give RESTORE a try. "I was so tired of just masking the symptoms," she told me. "I wanted to get to the root of the problem." Through a personalized combination of dietary changes, targeted therapies, and lifestyle adjustments, Jenny experienced remarkable progress.

"I can walk without pain again," she said, her face beaming with joy. "I'm even back to gardening, something I thought I'd never be able to do again!" While individual results may vary, Jenny's story shows that a comprehensive approach can make a world of difference in managing and relieving neuropathy symptoms.

ACTION STEP: Get Your Neuropathy Relief Stretch Handbook. **Master 11 Key Stretches** from Home To *Retrain Your Nerves and Regain Your Life.*

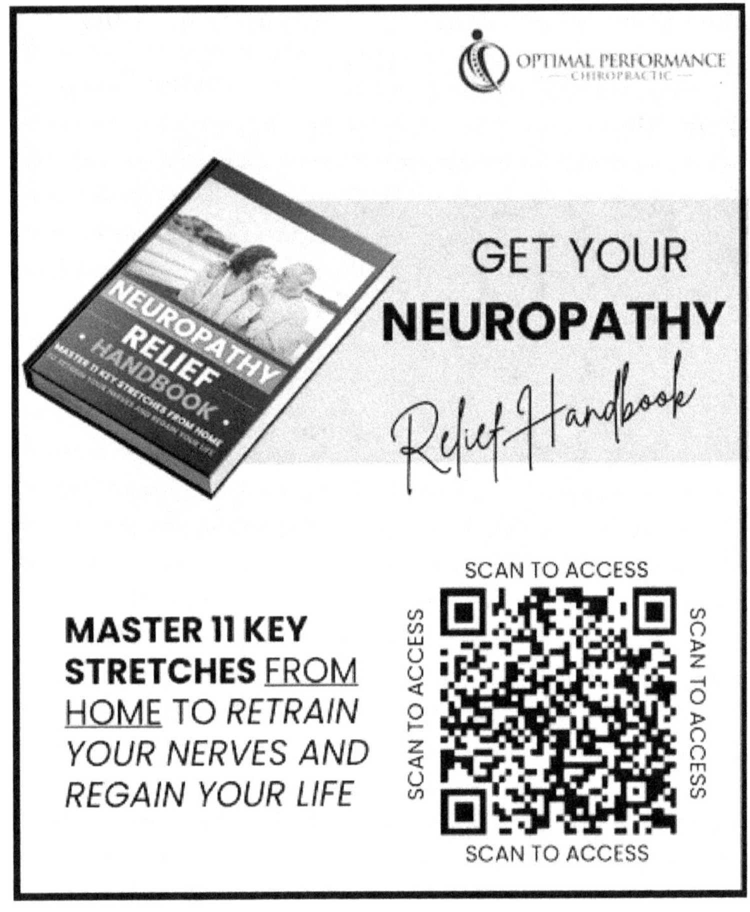

Unlock Your Path to Neuropathy Relief Now: Dial (951) 405-8868 to Speak With Us Today!

11

———

THE RESTORE REVOLUTION

Beyond Pills and Procedures

Neuropathy is a complex condition that can be challenging to treat. Conventional medicine often relies on medications and procedures to manage symptoms, but these approaches often fall short. They may provide temporary relief, but they do not address the root causes of neuropathy.

The RESTORE neuropathy healing framework is a different approach. It's a holistic path that focuses on healing the body from the inside out. The body can heal itself naturally, and we work with our patients to create an environment that supports healing.

We've seen countless people transform their lives through RESTORE. Here are a few more examples:

- Michelle had been struggling with neuropathy for years. She was constantly in pain and had difficulty walking. After just a few weeks of following the RESTORE program, Michelle's pain was significantly reduced, and she was able to walk again without difficulty.

- Mike had lost all feeling in his feet and hands. He was at risk of developing serious complications, such as foot ulcers and infections. After following the RESTORE framework for several weeks, Mike regained feeling in his feet and hands. He is now able to live a full and active life.

- Mary had been diagnosed with diabetic neuropathy and was feeling disheartened after being told she would have to manage her symptoms for the rest of her life. She struggled with pain, numbness, and limitations that were impacting her quality of life. Determined to find a better way to manage her condition, she decided to try the RESTORE framework. After incorporating the program's holistic strategies, including dietary adjustments, specialized therapies, and customized exercises, Mary experienced a significant improvement in her symptoms. She's now able to live a much more active and fulfilling life, with greater comfort and less reliance on pain management.

** The results described in these testimonials are not typical. Individual results may vary.*

The benefits of the RESTORE neuropathy healing framework go beyond simply relieving symptoms. When you heal from neuropathy, you can expect to experience the following:

- Lasting relief from pain, numbness, and tingling
- Improved nerve function
- Increased circulation
- Reduced inflammation
- Improved sleep quality
- Increased energy levels
- A rejuvenated life

If you're ready to transition into the RESTORE neuropathy healing framework, call us at (951) 405-8868. We can't wait to meet you and help you live healthy, happy, and pain-free.

The Role of Cutting-Edge Tech in RESTORE

Anyone who knows me knows that I am an analytical thinker and constantly pursuing the latest and greatest. If there is a new supplement with groundbreaking research, I want it for me and my patients. If there is a new treatment modality that shows major success, I want it for me and my patients.

In pursuing optimal neuropathy care, embracing cutting-edge technologies has become integral to the RESTORE neuropathy healing framework. This section explores three transformative technologies – SoftWave therapy, Infrared and Red Light Therapy, and the Balance Tracking System (BTrackS) – each designed to provide non-invasive, personalized, and practical solutions for individuals grappling with neuropathy.

SoftWave Therapy

SoftWave therapy is part of the RESTORE neuropathy healing framework, and it is a non-invasive treatment that uses focused acoustic waves to stimulate cell growth and regeneration. These waves can penetrate deep into the tissue, reaching areas that are difficult to access with other treatments.

In the context of neuropathy, SoftWave therapy can help to:

- Increase blood flow to the nerves
- Reduce inflammation
- Stimulate nerve regeneration
- Promote tissue healing

SoftWave therapy can lead to a significant reduction in neuropathy symptoms, such as pain, numbness, and tingling. It's also safe and well-tolerated, with minimal side effects like mild swelling.

How SoftWave Therapy Works

SoftWave therapy works by delivering low-frequency acoustic waves to the affected area. These waves create micro-cavitation bubbles, which collapse and release energy. This energy stimulates the production of growth factors and other molecules that promote cell growth and regeneration.

It also helps to reduce inflammation and improve blood flow. Inflammation is a significant contributor to neuropathy, and by reducing inflammation, SoftWave therapy can help to create an environment that is more conducive to healing.

SoftWave therapy has been shown to be effective in treating neuropathy in many clinical trials. For example, one study found that it significantly reduced pain and improved nerve function in people with diabetic neuropathy. Another study found that it was effective in treating neuropathy caused by chemotherapy.

We've been using SoftWave therapy to treat hundreds of neuropathy patients, and we've seen impressive results. Many of our patients at Optimal Performance Chiropractic have reported significant reductions in pain and numbness, and some have even experienced complete remission of their symptoms.

I'm particularly excited about SoftWave therapy because it's a non-invasive and drug-free treatment, meaning it's a safe and effective option for patients of all ages and health conditions.

If you're struggling with neuropathy, I encourage you to contact us about SoftWave therapy. It may be a life-changing treatment for you.

Infrared and Red Light Therapy

Infrared and red light therapy, also known as photobiomodulation (PBM), is a non-invasive treatment that uses specific wavelengths of light to stimulate the body's natural healing processes. One of the key benefits of this therapy is its ability to increase angiogenesis, which is the formation of new blood vessels.

By stimulating angiogenesis, infrared and red light therapy may help increase blood flow to the affected areas. This increase in circulation can bring more oxygen and nutrients to the nerves, potentially promoting healing and aiding in the management of neuropathy symptoms.

In addition to increasing blood and lymphatic flow, infrared and red light therapy also stimulate the production of growth factors and other molecules that promote cell growth and regeneration. This can help to repair damaged nerves and promote the formation of new blood vessels.

How Infrared and Red Light Therapy Works

Infrared and red light therapy works by delivering different wavelengths of light into the skin without damaging it. Infrared light has a longer wavelength than red light, which allows it to penetrate deeper into tissue.

When infrared and red light are absorbed by cells, they stimulate a number of cellular processes, including:

- Increased production of ATP (adenosine triphosphate), which is the body's energy currency.
- Increased production of nitric oxide, a vasodilator that helps widen blood vessels.
- Increased production of growth factors and other molecules that promote cell growth and regeneration.

Several clinical studies have shown that infrared and red light therapy can effectively treat neuropathy. For example, one study found that exposure to infrared light can reduce chronic pain without any adverse effects. In one trial, red light therapy was used to treat incurable, persistent nerve pain arising from a spinal cord injury.

Infrared and red light therapy is also part of the RESTORE program, and many patients have also reported that their pain and numbness have decreased significantly. It is also a non-invasive and drug-free treatment. This means they are a safe and effective option for patients of all ages and health conditions.

Balance Tracking System (BTrackS)

Another essential technological tool we use is our Balance Tracking System or BTrackS for short. The

BTrackS was developed and studied at Oakland University near Detroit. It is a non-invasive, easy-to-use system that measures your balance and fall risk.

It works by measuring the movement of your center of pressure. Your center of pressure is the point where all of the forces acting on your body intersect. When you're standing still, your center of pressure should be in the center of your body. However, if you have neuropathy, your center of pressure may constantly sway, which can increase your risk of falling.

The BTrackS provides a score that indicates your fall risk compared to people of the same age and gender. This score can be used to track your progress over time as your body and nerves begin to heal and perform better.

The BTrackS is a valuable tool for neuropathy treatment because it can help to:

- Identify people who are at high risk of falling
- Track the progress of neuropathy treatment
- Develop individualized treatment plans to improve balance
- Prevent falls and reduce the risk of injuries

How the Balance Tracking System Works

The BTrackS consists of a force plate and a computer software program. To use it, you stand on the force plate and follow a series of instructions on the computer screen. The force plate measures the movement of your center of pressure, and the computer software program calculates your fall risk score.

If you are concerned about your fall risk, please get in touch with us about the Balance Tracking System (BTrackS).

Technology is essential to the RESTORE healing framework for neuropathy because it allows us to provide precise, personalized treatment plans for each patient. With the help of technology, we can identify the root cause of your neuropathy, track your progress, and ensure that you receive the most effective treatment possible.

Embracing Daily Shifts: Integrating the RESTORE Neuropathy Program into Your Life

Living with neuropathy often means navigating limitations and discomfort. The RESTORE program aims to empower you to reclaim control and experience lasting improvement by integrating its principles into your daily routine. In this section, we'll explore how to seamlessly blend the RESTORE program into your life, reaping the benefits it offers.

Understanding Daily Integration

Integrating the RESTORE program isn't about drastic changes; it's about incorporating small, sustainable shifts into your existing lifestyle. When practiced consistently, these adjustments become powerful building blocks for healing and improved well-being.

Examples of Daily Integration

- **Diet:** Embrace nourishing foods rich in essential nutrients to support nerve health. Consider incorporating simple changes, like adding leafy greens to your meals or swapping sugary drinks for water.
- **Exercise:** Implement gentle, targeted exercises recommended by your healthcare professional. Start with short walks or stretching routines, gradually increasing intensity and duration as you progress.
- **Stress management:** Explore techniques like mindfulness or deep breathing to calm your nervous system and reduce stress, a known contributor to neuropathy symptoms.

Investing in Your Well-being

While some program elements may incur costs, like therapeutic consultations or specific equipment, consider the potential benefits:

- **Reduced pain and improved quality of life:** Less pain means a more active and enjoyable life, potentially reducing long-term healthcare costs.
- **Empowerment and control:** Taking charge of your healing journey fosters a sense of control and well-being, improving your overall health outlook.
- **Prevention of complications:** Addressing neuropathy proactively can help prevent serious complications like falls or infections, saving healthcare costs down the line.

Taking Action

1. **Tailor to your needs.** Discuss the program with your healthcare professional to customize it to your specific condition and preferences.
2. **Find support.** Connect with communities or support groups for encouragement, shared experiences, and motivation.

3. **Track your progress.** Monitor your symptoms, energy levels, and overall well-being to measure improvement and celebrate small victories.
4. **Be patient and persistent.** Remember, lasting change takes time and dedication. Embrace the journey, celebrate progress, and don't give up on your path to well-being.

Remember: You are not alone on this journey. Integrating the RESTORE program into your daily life will unlock a powerful approach to managing neuropathy, reclaiming your active life, and experiencing the joy of feeling your best once again. Start your personal shift towards well-being, one empowered step at a time.

Building Your Healing Circle: Cultivating a Support System for RESTORE Participants

Living with neuropathy can feel isolating, but you don't have to navigate this path alone. Establishing a strong support system is a fundamental pillar of the RESTORE program, empowering you to thrive on your healing journey. Let's explore how to build a robust support network and reap its invaluable benefits.

The Power of Connection

Think of your support system as a healing circle – diverse voices and unwavering encouragement surrounding you. This circle can include:

- **The Optimal Performance Chiropractic Team:** At Optimal Performance Chiropractic, we're passionate about helping you achieve your best health. Our team of dedicated professionals, including doctors, case managers, and rehabilitation specialists, is here to support you every step of the way on your journey to better well-being.
- **Family and Friends:** Share your journey with loved ones. Their understanding, encouragement, and practical assistance can be invaluable.
- **Support Groups:** Connecting with others facing similar challenges creates a sense of community and understanding. Share experiences, learn from each other, and gain strength through collective journeys.
- **Peers on Your RESTORE Journey:** Connect with fellow RESTORE participants through online forums or local gatherings. Sharing experiences, celebrating milestones, and

offering mutual support fosters a powerful bond and motivation.

Beyond Comforting Words

The benefits of a robust support system extend far beyond emotional encouragement:

- **Enhanced adherence:** Sharing goals and challenges with your support network fosters accountability, increasing your commitment to the program.
- **Personalized guidance:** Family and friends can offer practical support, adapting tasks or assisting with activities during challenging periods.
- **Information and resources:** Fellow participants and support groups can share valuable insights, success stories, and recommended resources related to neuropathy management.
- **Reduced stress and anxiety:** Feeling understood and supported reduces emotional burdens, easing stress and fostering a positive mindset conducive to healing.

Building Your Circle

1. **Start small.** Initially, reach out to close friends, family, or healthcare professionals you trust.
2. **Expand horizons.** Explore online forums, local support groups, or communities connected to RESTORE or relevant organizations.
3. **Be open and communicative.** Share your needs, challenges, and goals with your support system, encouraging open communication and understanding.
4. **Offer support in return.** Show your appreciation by actively listening, offering emotional support, and connecting others with helpful resources.
5. **Remember, it's a journey.** Cultivating a strong support system takes time and effort. Be patient, express gratitude, and nurture these connections for lasting benefits.

Your support system is a vital force in your healing journey. By building a diverse and supportive circle, you unlock a powerful source of encouragement, information, and motivation, empowering you to navigate challenges, celebrate victories, and reclaim your vibrant life.

The RESTORE program is here to support you every step of the way. Reach out, build your healing circle, and let's start your journey towards wellness together.

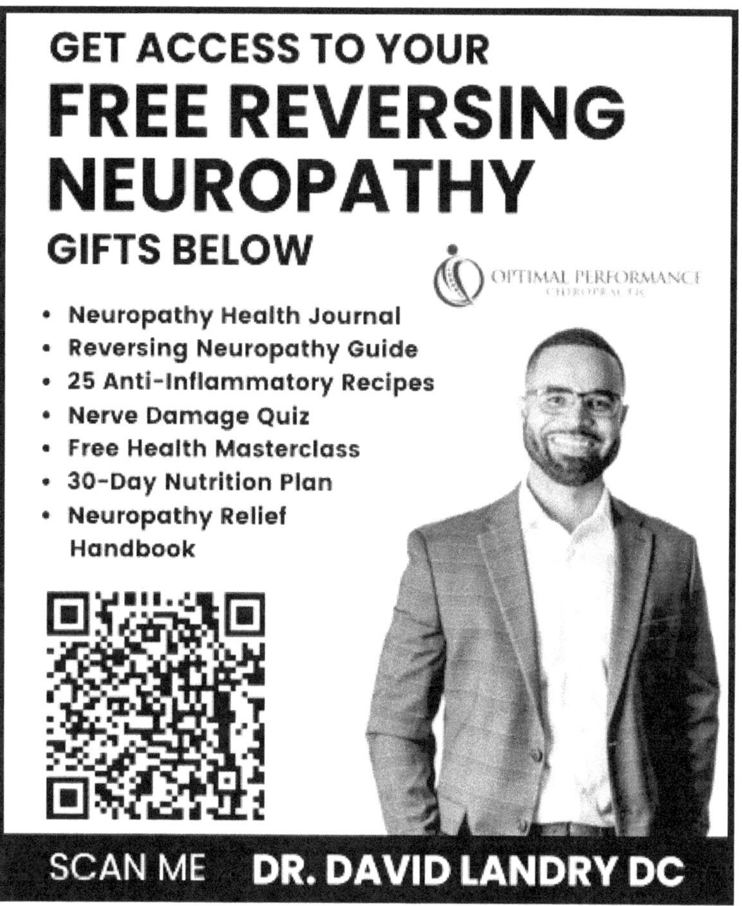

Unlock Your Path to Neuropathy Relief Now: Dial (951) 405-8868 to Speak With Us Today!

12

YOUR PATH TO PAIN-FREE LIVING STARTS NOW: THE RESTORE JOURNEY

I vividly recall a patient, let's call her Emily, who walked into my office with a cane, her face etched with worry. She'd been struggling with neuropathy for years, and the pain and numbness in her legs had progressed to the point where even short walks were excruciating.

"Doctor," she confessed, her voice trembling slightly, "I'm afraid I'm going to end up in a wheelchair. I just want to be able to play with my grandkids again without being in constant pain."

Emily was determined to regain her mobility and independence, and she embraced the RESTORE program with unwavering dedication. She diligently followed her personalized nutrition plan, consistently engaged in therapeutic exercises, and actively practiced stress management techniques.

Her commitment paid off. Month by month, I watched as Emily blossomed. Her pain gradually diminished, the numbness subsided, and her strength returned. The day she confidently walked into my office, cane-free, with a radiant smile illuminating her face, was a true testament to the power of perseverance and a holistic approach to healing. Of course, individual results can vary, and Emily's success isn't a guarantee for all patients. But her journey underscores the profound potential for healing when we address the root causes of neuropathy and empower our bodies to heal.

And now, it's your turn. Congratulations on making it this far in the book! Your dedication to relieving your neuropathy is truly inspiring. You now understand the complexities of this condition, the pitfalls of quick fixes, and the potential for true healing through the RESTORE method. But knowledge without action is like a seed unplanted – it holds potential but bears no fruit. Are you ready to cultivate that potential and see real change in your life?

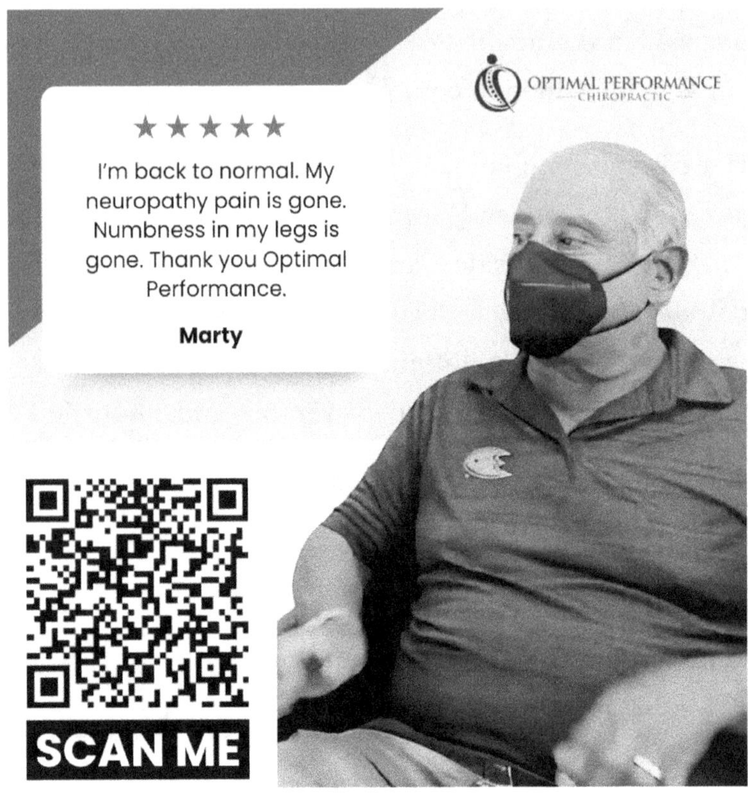

The 3 Secrets to Relieving Neuropathy Naturally

Join our free "3 Secrets to Relieving Neuropathy Naturally" online masterclass, where you'll discover the latest scientific evidence on how natural treatments can help you heal.

In this 30-minute masterclass, we'll cover the three breakthrough secrets to healing neuropathy:

1. **Oxygen and Angiogenesis** - Discover their potent synergy and how it rekindles healing, fostering new blood vessel growth to address the vital needs of nerve tissue and revive well-being.

2. **Inflammatory Regulation** - Unlock the secrets of reigniting healing and fostering new blood vessel growth while understanding the crucial difference between acute and chronic inflammation and its profound implications for neuropathy.

3. **Ignite Nerve Healing** - Learn the dynamic collaboration of the central and peripheral nervous systems and uncover tailored strategies for comprehensive healing.

We'll also show you how to use diet, exercise, and other holistic methods to restore nerve function and improve your overall well-being.

And, we'll take a holistic, whole-body approach to healing, addressing the root causes of neuropathy, such as spinal misalignments, compressed nerves, and impaired circulation.

Here are just a few more things that you'll learn at this free masterclass:

- The 4 common types of neuropathy
- The key to healing neuropathy
- The hidden root cause of neuropathy
- Top inflammatory triggers
- Strategies to reduce inflammation
- The power of neural stimulation
- And so much more!

Don't miss your chance to find the treasure of pain-free living. This masterclass is like a treasure map, with targeted, hands-on strategies to help you achieve your goal faster. But more than just physical relief, this can help you transform your entire life. Imagine being free from the prison of neuropathy and able to live confidently and to the fullest!

So go ahead and sign up for the free "3 Secrets to Relieving Neuropathy Naturally" masterclass today to discover the path to a pain-free life. Your RESTORE neuropathy breakthrough starts here. Sign up by scanning the code below.

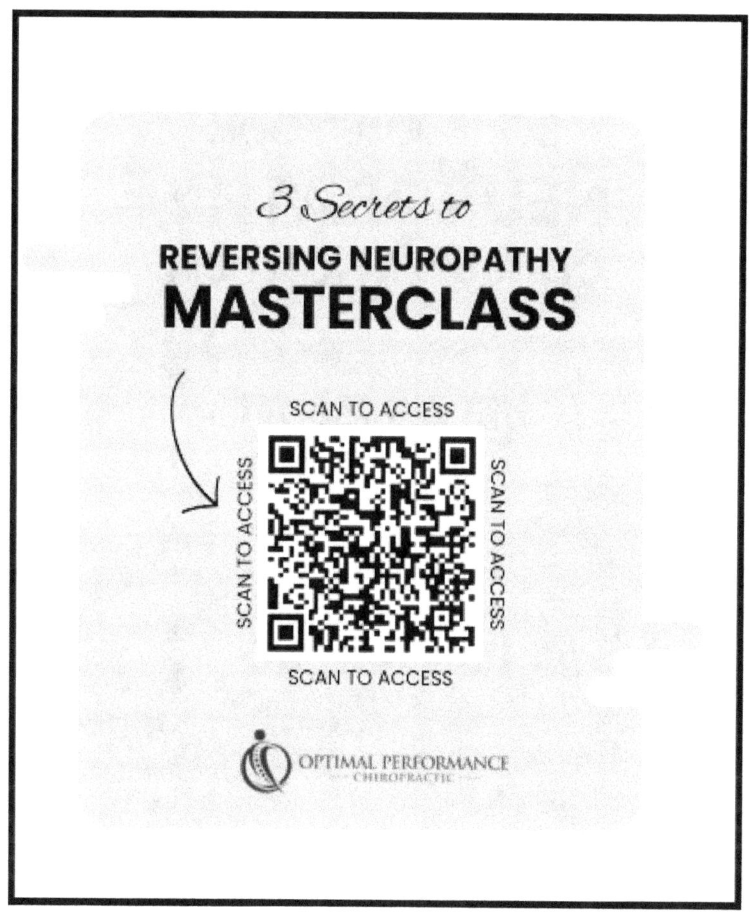

ACTION STEP: Want Help Now? Claim Your Private 1-on-1 Consultation Right Now: Find Relief The Natural Way: Relieve Neuropathy Pain Without Harmful Meds or Procedures!

Disclaimer: *This consultation is for informational purposes only and does not guarantee results. Every patient's journey is unique, and results may vary.*

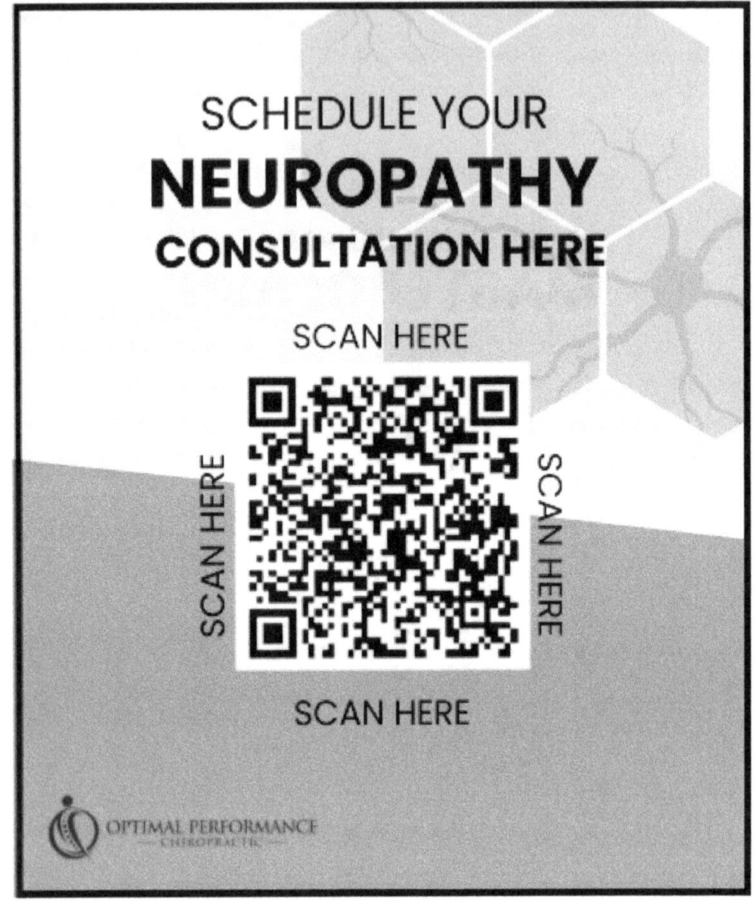

Thank you for taking the time to read "Relieving Neuropathy With RESTORE: Your Ultimate Guide to Conquering Neuropathy." We hope this book has empowered you with knowledge, hope, and a clear path toward reclaiming your life from the grip of neuropathy. Remember, you are not alone in this journey. The team at Optimal Performance Chiropractic is here to support you every step of the way. We are passionate about helping individuals like you find lasting relief and rediscover the joy of living without pain. We look forward to the opportunity to meet you, hear your story, and guide you on your personalized path to healing. Don't hesitate to reach out and take the first step towards a brighter, pain-free future. Your journey to wellness begins now!

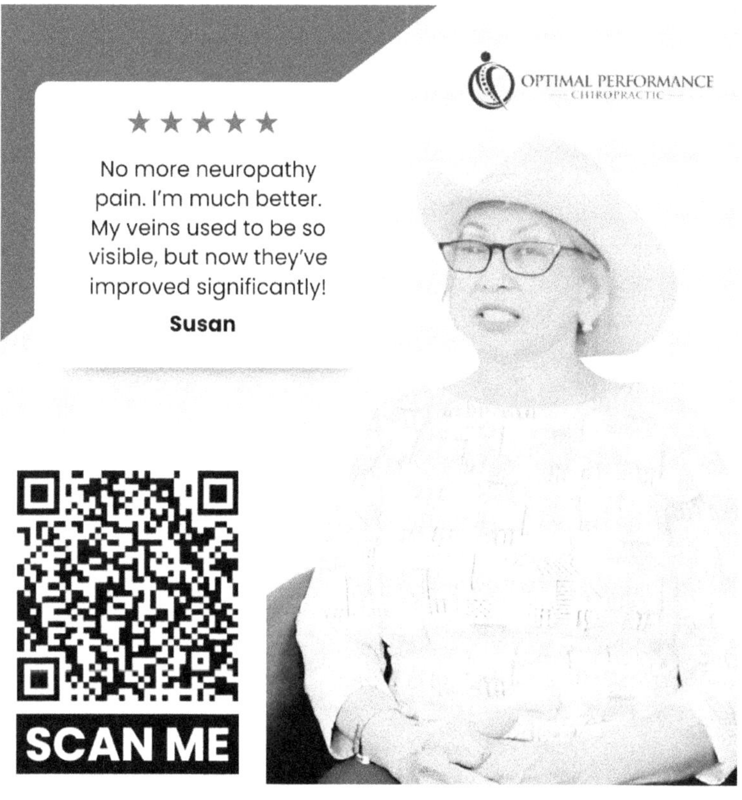

SOURCES

- McKinley-Barnard et al. Combined L-citrulline and glutathione supplementation increases the concentration of markers indicative of nitric oxide synthesis. Journal of the International Society of Sports Nutrition (2015) 12:27.
- Kochman AB, Carnegie DE, Burke TJ. Symptomatic Reversal of Peripheral Neuropathy in Patients with Diabetes. Journal of the American Podiatric Medical Association. 2002;92:125-130.
- Prendergast JJ, Miranda G, Sanchez M. Improvement of Sensory Impairment in Patients with Peripheral Neuropathy. Endocrine Practice. 2004;10:24-30.
- Leonard DR, Farooqi MH, Myers S. Restoration of Sensation, Reduced Pain, and Improved Balance in Subjects with Diabetic Peripheral Neuropathy; A Randomized, Double Blind, Placebo Controlled Study. Diabetes Care. 2004;27:168-172.
- Kochman AB. Monochromatic Infrared Photo Energy and Physical Therapy for Peripheral Neuropathy: Influence on Sensation, Balance and Falls. Journal of Geriatric Physical Therapy. 2004;27:16-19.
- Harkless L, DeLellis S, Burke TJ. Improved Foot Sensitivity and Pain Reduction in Patients with Peripheral Neuropathy after Treatment with Monochromatic Infrared Photo Energy-MIRE. Journal of Diabetes and Its Complications. 2006;20(2):81-87.
- Ammar, T. Monochromatic Infrared Photo Energy in Diabetic Peripheral Neuropathy. International Scholarly

Research Network (ISRN) Rehabilitation. 2012; Article ID 484307.

- Stanley Paul, Yuanlong liu, Robert McAlister The efficacy of monochromatic infrared photo-thermal energy therapy in rehabilitation: A pilot study report. Indian Journal of Physiotherapy and Occupational Therapy. January –March 2010, Vol.4, No.1

- Chen, Y et al. Extracorporeal shock wave therapy effectively prevented diabetic neuropathy. American Journal Transl Res 2015;7(12):2543-2560.

- Hausner T, Nógrádi A. The Use of Shock Waves in Peripheral Nerve Regeneration: New Perspectives? International Review of Neurobiology, 2013. Volume 109

- Schuh, C. M. A. P., Hercher, D., Stainer, M., Hopf, R., Teuschl, A. H., Schmidhammer, R., & Redl, H. Extracorporeal shockwave treatment: A novel tool to improve Schwann cell isolation and culture. Cytotherapy 2016, 18(6), 760–770.

- Hausner, T. et al. Improved rate of peripheral nerve regeneration induced by extracorporeal shock wave treatment in the rat. Experimental Neurology 2012, 236(2), 363–370.